stress

exercise plans to
improve your life

debbie lawrence and sarah bolitho

Other books in the *Exercise Your Way to Health* series:

Back Pain
Arthritis
Type 2 Diabetes
Osteoporosis
Depression

stress

exercise plans to improve your life

debbie lawrence and sarah bolitho

A & C Black • London

Note

Whilst every effort has been made to ensure that the content of this book is as technically accurate and as sound as possible, neither the authors nor the publishers can accept responsibility for any injury or loss sustained as a result of the use of this material.

Published in 2011 by A&C Black Publishers Ltd
36 Soho Square, London W1D 3QY
www.acblack.com

Copyright © 2011 Debbie Lawrence and Sarah Bolitho

ISBN 978 1 4081 3180 0

A CIP catalogue record for this book is available from the British Library.

Acknowledgements
Cover photograph © Shutterstock

Exercise photographs © Tom Croft

Inside photographs © Shutterstock except for those on pages xii, 6, 20, 29, 56 and 102 © Getty Images

Illustrations by Tom Croft

Designed by James Watson

Commissioned by Charlotte Croft

This book is produced using paper that is made from wood grown in managed, sustainable forests. It is natural, renewable and recyclable. The logging and manufacturing processes conform to the environmental regulations of the country of origin.

Typeset in 8.25pt Trade Gothic on 12pt by Saxon Graphics Ltd, Derby

Printed and bound in China by RR Donnelley South China Printing Co.

contents

acknowledgements

Writing, teaching and learning are my passions, so the opportunity to write this book brings great pleasure (a pleasant stress) and I am thankful to Charlotte Croft of A&C Black for asking me to contribute to the *Exercising Your Way to Health* series.

I give thanks to the 'ups, downs and plateaus' of life and living that I have experienced because they have made me the ever-evolving person that I am; and that we all are.

Special thanks to the 'ups' of life; from the part of me (my inner child) that likes them the most.

Special thanks to my partner, Joe, who, like a diamond, adds a sparkle to my life.

Thanks also to my Mum and Dad and brother for being part of my life!

I also give thanks to my co-writer, Sarah, who has combined her own wealth of experience with mine, to co-create this book.

Debbie Lawrence

To my father who has instilled in me a sense of honour and ethics that have supported me through many a stressful situation. He taught me that thinking slowly, talking calmly and looking at situations rationally are more productive than over-reacting. Thank you for everything, Dad, but most of all for your unconditional love.

To my children, Lucie, Danny and James, who, over the years, have provided me with much of the experience I needed to write this! You are all very special and I cherish each day with you.

Thank you also to Debbie, with whom I have shared the experience of writing this book – a welcome challenge!

Sarah Bolitho

The publishers would like to thank the David Lloyd Gym in Cardiff and Debbie Lawrence, Mary Sheppard, Jenny Burns, Rob Burns, Ben Burns, Mary Sparks and Paul Conway for their kind assistance with the photo-shoot.

foreword

Stress is, of course, part of our everyday life. All biological functions require a stimulus; hunger and thirst, for instance, are regular stressors that provoke the essential reactions of eating and drinking. Our fight or flight response, by which the body is instantly prepared for physical activity in the face of potential danger, has been a major factor in human survival for millennia.

However, in our less primitive, more industrialised society, physical action in the face of threat and pressure is often impossible. An impoverished single mother, receiving yet another bill, cannot simply attack the postman; a driver caught in a traffic jam and late for an important meeting cannot simply leave his car and jog to the office. Under these circumstances, the stresses are not released and, over time, they can lead to serious health problems including high blood pressure, heart disease, sleep disturbance and bowel disorders.

Learning to manage stress appropriately and to react to it in a less-damaging fashion is a vital skill of modern living, and using exercise as the tool is the perfect biological response. This clear guide on specific exercise programmes designed to help you cope with stress is written by two very experienced professionals in the field; it is an excellent means of both prevention of ill-heath and promotion of wellness. I recommend it to anyone who has ever felt stressed!

Dr C P Crosby MA (Oxon), FFSEM (UK), FFSEM (I), MB BS (Lond), LRCP MRCS Consultant in Sport and Exercise Medicine

introduction

The chances are that if you have picked up this book you want to know more about stress, how it affects your body and how you can manage or reduce your own stress levels. Perhaps you are concerned about your health because you are using other habits (alcohol, drugs, medication and/or cigarettes) to manage your stress? Well done! This is your first step in taking positive action to help yourself.

This book provides a simple overview explaining how stress levels can build up and the impact they have on our health. It is also full of valuable lifestyle tips and exercise ideas to help you make changes to your own stress levels and cope with stress.

Start exercising your way to health now!

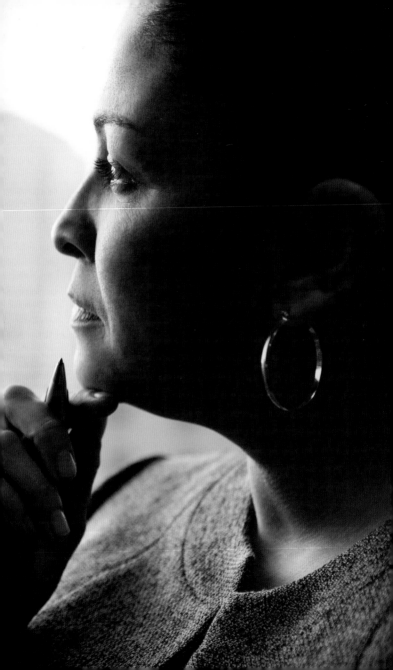

part

1

understanding stress

> > **What is stress?**

Although most of us will feel stressed or under pressure at some point in our life, stress is not actually an easy thing to define. Stress is a psychological condition that influences how we feel, think about and respond to the events, demands and challenges in our daily lives, and affects our perception of our ability to cope with these demands and experiences.

Life provides us with many potential *stimuli* or *stressors* both big and small: the work we do, the state of the economy, paying our bills, our relationships with friends and family, the way we think about ourselves, queuing in a supermarket, driving in traffic, world peace, exams, whether we take enough exercise, our habits, getting married or divorced … The list of potential stressors is endless and will change at different times throughout our lives.

However, not all stress is bad – we need some stimuli to function and to develop. It is when we are overwhelmed with stimuli or are less able to cope with them that stress takes over. It is a bit like watching a film: if it has a very complicated plot our minds have to work hard to try to make sense of it so we may leave the cinema with a sense of frustration. Too simple and we may get so bored that we fall asleep. If we'd read the reviews or the plot line before going to the cinema, we might have had a clearer idea of the plot and been able to follow it – or decided it wasn't for us and chosen a different film instead. The reviews would have been a useful source of information, or 'resource'.

Coping with stress requires us to use our own resources – things that help us cope with the demands of life. They are often simple habits such as taking a breath before we speak, spending five minutes a day in quiet reflection, getting tomorrow's clothes or bag ready the night before, having a list of due dates for insurance and bills, and so on. Resources may also be more complex or may come from other sources such as visiting a therapist or learning new skills to help with our personal development; or they may be from the people around us such as babysitters, parents, friends and family, who already do, or would like to, help out.

So what are your existing resources? Try taking a pen and paper and writing them down, using the resources log in the appendices on page 000. On one side put your resources, and on the other describe how you use them. For example:

Resource
- Keeping close to my family
- My computer
- Being organised with paperwork

Uses
- Advice and emergencies
- Online shopping / banking
- Paying bills on time

If our coping resources are strong and we use them, we are better equipped to recognise and deal with unwanted stress, but if they are weak or we are reluctant to use them, we may not be able to identify when we are stressed or be able to cope with it. Developing these coping resources is like learning anything – practise, practise, practise! The more we do something, the better we get at it so the more we take a deep breath before we react in a stressful situation, the easier it is to do and it will eventually become automatic – which is good.

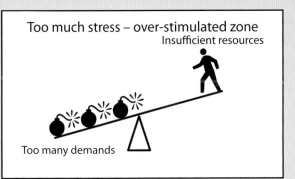

Too much stress – over-stimulated zone

Insufficient resources

Too many demands

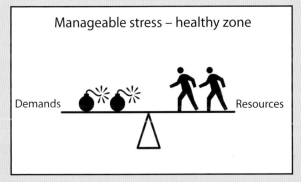

Manageable stress – healthy zone

Demands

Resources

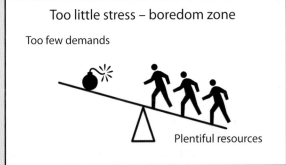

Too little stress – boredom zone

Too few demands

Plentiful resources

Stress balance: your demands and resources need to balance to keep you stress-free.

On the other hand, this also means that each time we react in a bad way, such as getting angry, we get better at getting angry. Not so good. Having said this, anger is a natural emotion and should not be blocked, but it needs to be channelled and expressed in a helpful way.

> The key thing to bear in mind is that a certain amount of stress is healthy and normal! The right balance of stress and coping resources can help us to develop ourselves in our work, home or social lives. It can teach us to accept and enjoy challenges and know when we need to say no or accept help.

> ## PERCEPTION

This brings us nicely to another way of looking at stress – as either a good thing or a bad thing. We are born to different families in different cultures with different social, educational and financial backgrounds; each of us has our own unique experience and view of life. Each of these factors affects how we respond to the things that happen in our lives and how we believe we are able to cope. Something you may find stressful (such as starting a new job or taking an exam) may be a pleasure or positive stressor to me, while what I perceive as unacceptably stressful may be an exciting challenge to you.

Most of us have a tendency to see stress as a bad thing, focusing on the things that could go wrong, instead of seeing it as something that may be positive for us and from which we can learn. It is not easy to change the way we think about stress, but by training ourselves to look at things in a positive way (as well as negative!) we may see opportunities or advantages that help us get through it or give us the strength to say 'not now'.

Sometimes saying yes to everything means others think we are coping well or want more work – or don't have enough to do! Despite what the authors continue to learn and know about their own stress, even they sometimes end up doing this! When this happens it helps to remember that you are not infallible and celebrate this 'realness' in yourself.

> ### Paul and Tim

Paul was already overwhelmed with 'important' tasks from his boss when he was given another 'urgent' task. He accepted the work without comment, which resulted in him becoming so stressed that he fell ill and had to take time off work, which caused him even more stress.

Another colleague, Tim, in a similar situation, went back to his boss with all the tasks he had on his plate and said, 'If you want me to do this new task, which of these can I put on hold?' His boss reacted by saying he had no idea how much Tim was already doing and not only gave the new task to someone else but arranged an assistant to help Tim with his current workload.

There are some life experiences that most of us would perceive and experience as negative (for example, someone close to us dying, being diagnosed with a long-term or serious illness, separation or divorce, or financial troubles). In these circumstances, we need to gather and build our resources and make it easier to get through them by asking for help, keeping our health in good condition or seeking support.

> INNER AND OUTER RESOURCES

Some of us have what we call *external* resources. Friendship and family are important – someone to talk to when things are tough. However, we may still believe we're unable to cope because our *inner* resources (like self-belief, self-esteem, self-confidence and thinking habits) may lead us to believe we are not up for challenge.

Alternatively, some of us may have fewer external resources (no savings, or family living a long way away) but our inner resources are strong enough to help us believe we are able to cope. We know we can handle whatever life deals us, because, ultimately, we have to.

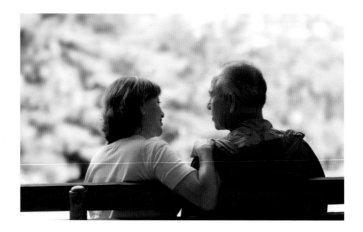

Most of us just need a little help to see our inner strength and power. This is where counselling and other therapeutic remedies can be useful ways of helping us during times of stress. They offer somewhere for us to take the time to learn to build these inner resources like self-esteem, self-confidence, self-efficacy (our inner belief that we can do a particular task) and our belief in our ability to handle all, or most, situations.

Louise

Any situation has the potential to become negatively stressful if we feel we're 'unable to cope'. Sometimes we are in a good place and feel that we can manage but at other times events can overwhelm us.

Many years ago Louise had to move home as a result of divorce. The combination of three very young children, a sense of loss from the breakdown of her marriage and having to cope with the financial and legal stuff made it a very stressful period; she became quite ill and ended up seeing herself in a negative way. Recently she moved again, this time out of choice, and the process was much less stressful, as she perceived it to be a positive and exciting thing. Same event, same stressors but two very different outcomes.

>> What are the causes of stress?

There are lots of different events that can contribute to stress. It would be impossible to go through life without encountering some of them – and who would want to? Especially since 'stressors' can also be very important and pleasurable things like getting married or going on holiday.

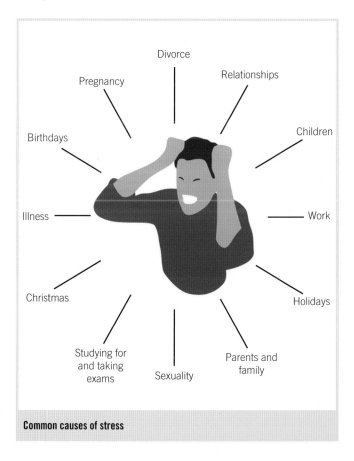

Common causes of stress

There are also numerous and arguably less significant life experiences that can contribute to our feeling stressed, such as getting a bad haircut, queuing at the supermarket, someone being rude to us or our washing machine breaking down.

> CATEGORIES OF STRESSORS

Stressors fall into different categories. For example, physical stress may result from pregnancy or being unwell or overtired. We may also be psychologically stressed by bullying, rudeness or prejudice, while our emotions may come under fire from relationship problems or if someone calls us a horrible name (verbal abuse) or even if we get a bad haircut, which affects how we see ourselves.

There are also deeper endemic, or far-reaching, causes of stress. These are often things over which we have less control – global problems such as the environment, climate change, the financial crisis or the presence or threat of war. Things closer to home but equally out of our control, including work and relationships, affect us socially. Pollution or noise around us may affect our ability to cope with other stressors. Put all these together and our philosophical or spiritual self may be affected and start to question our values or sense of purpose.

The lists and categories of potential stressors are endless and will always be around, unless we lock ourselves away and become hermits. The key thing to remember is that, as the famous Shakespearean saying goes, 'there is nothing either good or bad, but thinking makes it so'.

> THINGS WE CANNOT CHANGE

In life there are many potential stressors over which we have no control – the 'givens' – and some of these are mentioned above: climate change, financial crisis, war. How we deal with these can have an impact on our overall stress levels so it is important to find a constructive solution to our concerns and do what we can within reason to help.

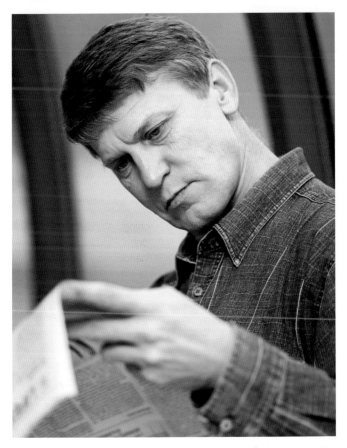

For example, there may be small ways we can reduce our own negative impact on our environment. We can recycle, switch off lights, pick up litter, cycle to work and choose organic products. However, it is unlikely that we can have a major impact on a national or international level without becoming high-ranking politicians or advisors – which brings a whole new source of stress! For some people, picking up a newspaper and reading about the latest flood or oil spill will cause real stress, because they feel powerless to change the situation. The problem seems like a personal responsibility.

But it's important to consider these givens as just that – given things that are out of our control on a large scale. Avoid allowing these to add more stress or worry to your life, particularly when there is little you can do, and focus on the changes and contributions you can make on a local or personal scale. And know that the little things can sometimes make a big difference. If you have ever tried to sleep with a dripping tap in the background which suddenly stops, you will know what we mean!

The Serenity Prayer

God, grant me the serenity to accept the things I cannot change,
The courage to change the things I can,
And the wisdom to know the difference.

Reinhold Niebuhr 1943

>> What effect does stress have on me?

As human beings we've evolved a lot since our hunter-gatherer days. Unfortunately, the way we respond in stressful situations has remained more primitive and less evolved. In the days when we lived in caves and had to hunt for our food and fight off or run from wild beasts, the 'fight or flight' response was a great asset (see box on page 11).

The body's response to stress is show on pages 12 and 13. Most of these effects are caused by the *sympathetic nervous system*, which acts as an accelerator and triggers the release of adrenaline and noradrenaline. These two chemicals act to speed up and/or improve efficiency of the systems shown in the figure, enabling us to cope with the stressor more effectively.

Once the initial stress has been dealt with or has passed, another system kicks in – the *parasympathetic nervous system*. This provides a 'braking' effect brought about by a chemical called acetylcholine, which acts to slow down the effects of the sympathetic nervous system and return us to a state of (relative) calm. During fight or flight this system becomes inactive, as its role is to save energy, assist digestion and protect against foreign bodies. If it kept working it would lead to the secretion of tears, saliva, mucus (from nose and throat) and gastric juice in the stomach and would compete with the muscles for blood, inhibiting the fight or flight response.

What is fight or flight?

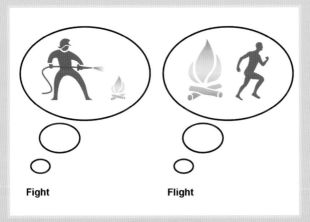

Fight   **Flight**

When we encounter a situation that makes us feel under pressure or stressed, our body stimulates the fight or flight reaction. Part of this is the release of chemicals such as adrenaline, noradrenaline and cortisol to help us deal with the threat.

Put simply, if we receive a stimulus – or fright – our bodies prepare themselves to attack (fight) or retreat (flight). So if we come across a large forest fire our bodies prepare instantly for flight to get away from it, while finding a small fire is more likely to create a fight response so we can put it out.

If were were indeed facing a forest fire, this reaction could save our lives. However modern life often means that we feel this primal response in situations where we cannot channel it – for instance, at work or in a traffic jam. Then the chemicals accumulate in the body; the long-term effects of this build-up are discussed on pages 14 to 16.

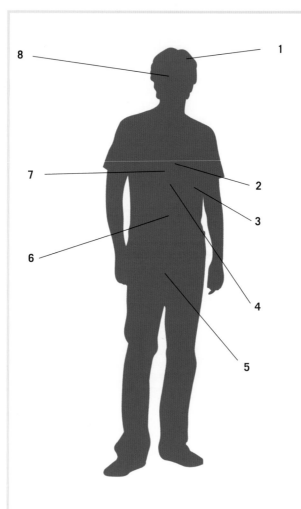

How the body responds to stress

1 The brain evaluates signals sent by your senses and decides what to do. Other parts of the brain add emotions such as fear, anger and excitement. Messages are sent via the nervous system to release hormones.

2 The airways widen and breathing rate increases and deepens to take in more oxygen and get rid of more carbon dioxide.

3 The body prepares for fight or flight by releasing two chemicals, adrenaline and noradrenaline, from the adrenal glands at the top of each kidney.

4 The liver releases glycogen (our main energy source) and fat into the bloodstream. They are carried to the working muscles and provide the energy needed for flight or flight.

5 Blood moves away from the sexual organs. Blood is also diverted away from the skin to prevent excessive bleeding while sweat is produced to keep the body cool.

The small blood vessels in the muscles (capillaries) widen to get more blood and oxygen to the muscles. Your muscles tense in preparation for fight or flight.

6 The digestive system slows down because blood diverts from the digestive system to provide more oxygen for the muscles.

7 Heart rate and blood pressure increase to get more blood and oxygen around the body and to the muscles that are preparing for flight or fight.

8 All the senses become more alert in response to the perceived threat:
- Sight improves
- Hearing sharpens
- Smells become more acute
- Taste heightens
- Touch becomes more sensitive
- Intuition heightens – the hairs on the back of your neck stand up
- Pain reactions numb to protect against injury

Since many of the stressors we experience in modern life are less physical and dangerous than those our ancestors had to deal with in the Stone Age, our response is often a static one; that is, while our bodies prepare us for either fight or flight in the old primitive way, we are not in a position to react with either. This, together with the fact that a great many of us are not achieving healthy levels of physical activity which would act as an appropriate outlet, means that the effects of stress can accumulate and build up in the body.

> This is one of the reasons why getting up and doing some exercise is so helpful for managing some of the signs and symptoms of stress. It uses your body's stress response efficiently and returns the body to a more balanced state. It doesn't need to be an aggressive form of exercise. You can reach for your walking shoes or your boxing gloves – whatever works for you!

>> What are the effects of long-term stress?

The build-up of adrenaline and noradrenaline over time increases heart rate, blood pressure and breathing rate. Blood supply is diverted from the digestive system to the muscles, which tense up ready for action. Over time, the body remains in a perpetually 'semi-aroused' state that results in increased heart rate and blood pressure, muscle tension, poor digestion and a sense of edginess.

Long-term exposure to stress can make us more susceptible to and at risk of other health problems, such as:

- High blood pressure
- High cholesterol
- Coronary heart disease
- Osteoporosis
- Depression
- Anxiety disorders

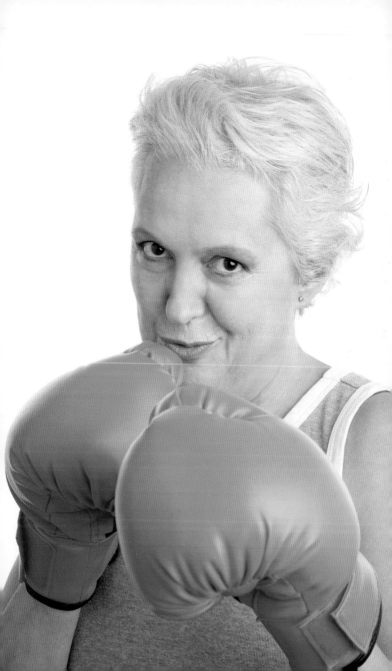

- Irritable bowel syndrome
- Some cancers
- Alcohol-related problems
- Eating disorders

THE HEART AND CIRCULATION

The combination of excess blood sugar and fats released during stressful times to provide energy may contribute to damage and furring of the artery walls (atherosclerosis), which is one of the most significant risks for coronary artery disease.

THE BONES AND JOINTS

Too much cortisol in the system is not good for the bones as it slows down the production of new bone cells, which increases the risk of osteoporosis and fractures.

Being stuck at the desk or in the car or slumped in front of the TV also means we are more inactive, which affects the joints as they need movement to keep healthy. Backache is particularly common in people who experience a lot of stress.

THE IMMUNE SYSTEM

Part of the reaction to stress is the activation of hormone release by certain parts of the brain and nervous system (the pituitary and adrenal glands) and over longer periods of stress these become more dominant and trigger increased levels of adrenaline, noradrenaline and cortisol to supply energy. It also leads to increased levels of chemicals such as insulin in the body, which may affect insulin resistance and fat usage and result in weight gain around the waist.

Unfortunately, these higher levels of hormones (chemicals) also suppress the immune system which makes us more susceptible to illness or disease such as colds and flu. It also appears to make us more at risk of autoimmune conditions such as rheumatoid arthtitis, lupus and chronic fatigue syndrome as well as increasing our risk of certain cancers. A less effective immune system can also affect the body's healing ability, which means it may take longer to recover from illness or for injuries or wounds to heal.

THE RESPIRATORY SYSTEM

Long-term stress may induce and increase the symptoms of asthma and other respiratory conditions.

THE DIGESTIVE SYSTEM

The stress reaction means that the digestive system becomes suppressed, which may lead to disorders such as constipation, diarrhoea and irritable bowel syndrome, or other unwelcome effects such as flatulence.

THE REPRODUCTIVE SYSTEM

Levels of the male hormone testosterone (and the female version, androstenedione) can increase when we feel secure – when we experience feelings of power, control, dominance or success in a particular situation. Levels of sex hormones can play a key role in influencing our social behaviour and relationships.

Suppression of the reproductive system can lead to a lack of menstruation in women (amenorrhea), impotence in men and loss of libido in both genders, and these are likely to cause stress and other problems in relationships.

WEIGHT AND DIABETES RISK

Long-term stress can have an effect on managing blood sugar levels and may be linked to adult-onset diabetes.

Fats are released by the liver to provide a readily available source of energy for dealing with the stressor but are likely to be stored in fat cells if the anticipated flight or flight does not happen, leading to an increase in weight and fat levels, particularly around the waist.

> > How do I know I'm stressed?

Some signs of stress are obvious but some are hidden. There are certain signs and symptoms of stress with which we are more familiar, and which are perhaps easier to spot. Many of these, however, may come on over a period of time which means they may not be so obvious to us. Others around us may notice them more quickly, so talk to family and friends and try to take on board their concerns.

The good news is that it's often when we experience a *build-up* of the different signs and symptoms and the accumulation of chemicals that we stop, take notice, become aware of our stress and take steps towards dealing with it.

Look at the MOT questionnaire on page 23 and be honest with yourself – are you answering 'always' and 'frequently' more often than you would like? Are you being affected mentally, physically or emotionally by stress, and is it having an impact on your behaviour? If your answer is yes, then you may be experiencing considerable stress. Depending on how you are feeling, it might be time to make a change that can help you take control of your stress – see Parts 2 and 3 for guidance – or it might be time to visit your doctor to discuss things.

Remember that this book is not designed to replace a medical check-up or advice offered by your GP or health professional. It can help you manage your stress, but if things are very bad it is a good idea to talk to your doctor.

A formal diagnosis of chronic stress depends on a mix of complex factors and does require you to be honest with yourself and your doctor about all your symptoms – physical and mental.

It is important to recognise and deal with stress if it becomes constant or if there are insufficient periods of calm between periods of high stress. If left unchecked it can all too easily lead to more significant mental health problems such as anxiety or depression.

Prescription medication

For many people, one of the first steps towards better stress management may be prescribed medication. This can be a significant factor in coping when everything seems to be overwhelming, but only you and your doctor should decide if this is the best route for you.

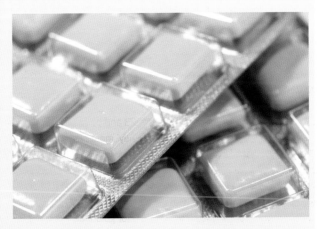

You may be reluctant to go down this road or you may feel that you are not 'that bad' yet. But even if you do need the support of medication it doesn't have to be long term and may give you enough help to cope in the short term, and provide you with the chance to be able to practise some of the lifestyle techniques outlined in this book, which will help in the long term.

Medicine and exercise

There may be side effects to any medication, particularly in the early stages, so if you are experiencing these it is advisable to discuss becoming more active with your doctor. However, as long as you take activity slowly and build up gradually, these effects should not prevent you from doing some basic exercise.

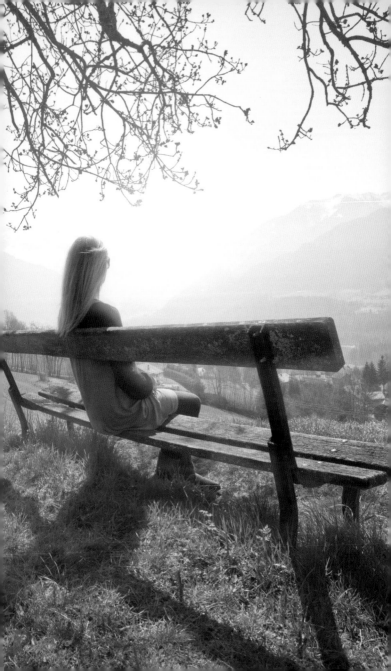

part

2

helping yourself to health

>> Where to start?

Making changes to your life can seem daunting, especially if you are already feeling stressed and under pressure. This section is designed to help you take the small simple steps that lead to big results.

You need to consider first what you can actually do to help yourself. Taking the opportunity to help yourself will give you back some personal power and will help you to regain control, rather than letting stress control you. What follows is a simple four-step strategy to assist you.

> STEP 1. TAKE THE MOT
The first step in this process is to take a look at yourself and recognise your own stress levels. On pages 23 to 25 you will find a detailed MOT questionnaire. This is designed to help you work out exactly how stressed you are, and what effect this is having on you right now.

Have a look through, and tick the answers that apply to you. Of course these might vary from week to week, but will still give you an overview of your current stress levels.

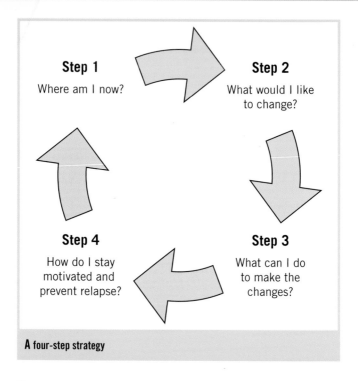

A four-step strategy

The more *always* and *frequently* responses you tick, the more risk factors you have and the more changes you need to make to start reducing your stress levels. If you have mainly answered *occasionally* and *never*, you are probably aware of your stress and have some coping strategies in place.

Go back and look at your answers to see which categories most of them fall into: mental, emotional, physical, behaviour. This may highlight a particular area that needs your attention.

Don't feel worried if it's clear that your stress levels are very high. Completing the MOT questionnaire and being honest with yourself is the first step on the road to taking control. Now you know what is wrong, the next step is to decide what you want to change.

The MOT questionnaire				
MOT questionnaire	always	frequently	occasionally	never
Mental: Is your mind affected by?				
Irrational thoughts				
More than normal tiredness				
Poor decision-making				
Negative thoughts about yourself or others				
Unable to listen to others				
Putting things off till tomorrow				
Excessive self-criticism				
Focusing only on yourself				
Making mistakes				
Emotional: Do you feel?				
Sad				
Angry				
Depressed				
Scared				
Panic				
Irritable				
Bored				
Lonely				
Jealous				
Resentful				
Helpless				
Powerless				

MOT questionnaire	always	frequently	occasionally	never
Insecure				
Frustrated				
Lethargic				
Unfocused				
Tearful				
Anxious				
Hopeless				
Physical: Do you experience?				
Spots or skin disorders				
Shoulder tension				
Chest pain				
Increased heart rate				
Nervous indigestion				
Fast shallow breathing				
Upper back hunched				
Yawning or sighing a lot				
Increased blood pressure				
Abdominal pain				
Sexual difficulties				
Clenched jaw				
Menstrual disorders				
Flatulence				
Allergies				
Hair loss				
Dry mouth				
Tense forehead / headaches				

MOT questionnaire	always	frequently	occasionally	never
Behavioural: Are you?				
Eating more or less				
Drinking more stimulants (coffee, tea, etc.)				
Drinking more alcohol				
Smoking more				
Swearing more				
Exercising more or less				
More argumentative and aggressive				
Crying more				
Increased or decreased sexual libido				
Talking more				
Blinking more				
Foot tapping				
Cannot sit still				
Picking at skin				
Pulling or splitting hair				
Biting nails				
Grinding teeth				
Gripping hands				
Driving faster				

> ### STEP 2: SET GOALS AND TARGETS

The primary aim of this book is to promote your physical activity and exercise levels. However, it's important to look at your lifestyle and habits generally, as there are many factors that could be contributing to your stress levels and which you should consider changing. This could be anything from giving up smoking and taking more exercise to giving yourself ten minutes of peace and quiet a day.

Quiet space

Your quiet space can be real or virtual, but it needs to be somewhere where you can take a few minutes to help you move from 'work me' to 'home me'. This may be sitting in a corner of your home or garden that you particularly like, or a five-minute lie-down on the bed. It could be a short walk or ten minutes gardening – anywhere that gives you time alone.

If you know you're stressed but are not sure what goal to set yourself, then start by reading through the 'lifestyle focus' starting on page 31. This section covers some of the different areas where improvements can usually be made. Here are a few examples. Do any of them apply to you? If so, remember that these 'every day' things can be the cause of serious mental and physical stress:

- inactive lifestyle
- sedentary job
- no exercise
- smoking
- drinking too much
- caffeine overdose
- bad diet
- too many fizzy drinks
- too busy
- insomnia
- low self-esteem
- feel like a doormat
- can't say 'no' to extra work
- feel out of control

- no time for yourself
- critical of self and others

You may be overwhelmed by the quantity of things you want to change. Remember that it's usually best to focus on one or two small changes and do them well, rather than changing lots of things at one time.

Set yourself SMART targets

- **S**pecific: What are you going to do?
- **M**easurable: How will you know and check you have done it?
- **A**chievable: Is it manageable for you? Will you do it?
- **R**ealistic: Is your target realistic?
- **T**ime-framed: Is there a time frame?

> STEP 3: TAKE ACTION

It's great to say you want to eat more healthily, sleep better, give up smoking, exercise more … But how do you achieve this? Being specific is key. Breaking your goal down into small, easy-to-achieve steps makes it much more realistic and helps you get started. For example:

Goal: 'To take regular exercise' can be turned into a measurable target: 'to walk for 30 minutes on 5 days of this week.' This can be broken down further, so you goal becomes:

- I will walk for 10 minutes after each meal.

Goal: 'To relax more' can become a measurable target: 'I will relax for 15 minutes when I get home from work.' This can be made more achievable by breaking it down to:

- I will go straight to the garden with a book when I get home; no TV, no housework, just a few minutes of 'me' time.

Goal: 'Not to get stressed at work' can become a measureable target: 'I will do some simple desk exercises for ten minutes every morning and afternoon.' This can become:

- I will set my phone to remind me to exercise at 10.30 and 3.30 every day.

It is also important to set a start date or time. You can always start next week, or tomorrow – but why not start right now? Making progress towards your goal has a very positive psychological effect, and will help you build up momentum.

> Carol was unhappy at work and in her relationship; she also lacked self-confidence. She knew she needed to make some changes in her life. Her GP referred her to counselling because she was experiencing stress and displaying symptoms of mild depression.
>
> She loved yoga and set a goal to start making time first thing in the morning for a short five-minute yoga practice. She didn't do this every day, but she did manage it on a couple of days of the week and it made a difference!
>
> 'I know this isn't changing everything in my life, but it is making a difference to me. I feel better about myself and it is good to do something just for me and not be running around after everyone else. It may give me the courage to make some of the other changes that I need to make.'
>
> **Carol, aged 29**

> ## STEP 4: THE CARROT!
It is so easy to lose sight of all the positive steps you are taking and the changes you are making. For this reason, it's important to review your progress and notice everything that you *do*, rather than focusing on the

things you don't. There is no need to feel downhearted if you miss an exercise session or if you eat the wrong food or have too much to drink. The key to making changes is to allow yourself to do it gradually.

> If you slip up and relapse a lot, perhaps you have set your goal too high and it is not realistic? In this case, go back and check that your goal is SMART for you (see page 27).

MAKE A NOTE

It can really help to keep a record, focusing on the positive changes you make by recording them in a log. It is amazing how forgetful the mind can sometimes be about the positive things we do, particularly when we feel stressed and under pressure.

It's also a useful tool for analysing just what you do all day long. It might surprise you to realise that you're much more active than you think, or that you actually eat less or smoke less than you fear. On the other hand, it can help you to identify areas where you could do more. If you sit still all afternoon from 2pm to 5.30pm, for example, you could try to introduce a ten-minute walk or stretch each day at 3.30pm.

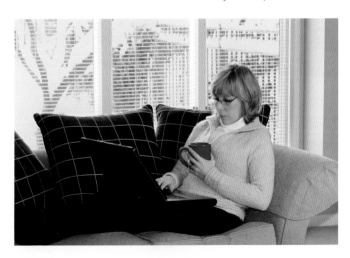

KNOW YOURSELF

Occasional slips are a natural part of the process of change and we can learn from them. Get to know yourself: be a student of your life and identify the danger signs. If you get down and demoralised when you are over-tired, try to get enough sleep each night. If you eat when you are stressed, keep healthy snacks to hand. If you can't resist smoking socially, stay away from people who smoke, at least during the early days of giving up. You can't always have a strategy to prevent slips though – learn to forgive yourself, and begin again.

> If you are pleased with your progress 80% of the time, then the odd 20% of 'naughty but nice' is fine. Don't be downhearted – remember that life is for living, and don't let guilt throw you off balance and ruin your efforts.

CATCH THE UNHELPFUL THOUGHT

The thoughts we have can affect the way we see ourselves and our achievements, our life and relationships. Unhelpful and negative thoughts can also decrease our motivation.

Simply spotting them is very useful. It allows us to think before we give in to their negative influence.

But how do you do this?

The trick is, whenever you find yourself thinking or speaking a negative thought ('I am no good', 'I can't do this'), call time out or shout 'stop'. Recognise the thought for what it is, then just let it go.

This is a technique that takes time and practice, but it does get easier. It increases an awareness of your own thought patterns and helps you break free from negative cycles.

MIND YOUR LANGUAGE

Notice the words you use to dictate your life experience. Use words that enable you take responsibility and be powerful, rather than words that disempower you and keep you low.

Don't use:

- I must
- I should
- I'll fail
- I can't
- It's not my fault

Do use:

- I want
- I choose
- I'll learn
- I can
- I can take responsiblity

>> # Lifestyle focus

The greatest changes you can make to improve your overall health and combat stress are simple yet effective. From taking time to focus on your breathing (page 000) to exercising for half an hour a day, there are lots of techniques to help you take control back.

We will talk about exercise in detail in Part 3, but there are many other ways to change your lifestyle for the better, from giving up smoking to finding some 'you' time. All of them play an important part in reducing the effects of stress.

Read through this section and see if any of the following areas are ones you'd like to change in your own life. This will help you set your goals and move forward in the four-step strategy described at the start of this section.

There are also some super-stress busters listed on page 000, designed to provide a quick-fix when you're feeling under pressure.

> **BEING MORE ACTIVE**

One of the most effective ways to use that fight or flight response in the way it was intended is by doing something physically active. This may help to give you a sense of control that assists in maintaining a balanced state of mind and body. The Chief Medical Officer's report 'At least five a week' (2004) recommends activity to help manage or reduce stress and to benefit mental health, and both the charity Mind and the Mental Health Foundation recommend physical activity to help reduce symptoms and risk of mental health problems.

You do not need to grab a pair of trainers and head out at 6am for an hour-long run (unless you want to, of course). Building activity into your everyday life is actually quite simple and once you have started to do this, you will feel the benefits very quickly.

Ideas for getting more active:

- Walk the dog
- Walk the kids to school
- Walk to the shops instead of taking the car
- Walk in your lunch hour
- Do the shopping for your neighbour
- Exercise at your desk
- Do some gardening
- Do the housework with vigour
- Walk up escalators
- Put on some music and move around
- Park your car further away from the office or supermarket
- Buy a Wii Fit or an exercise video
- Join a walking group like the Ramblers
- Get on the bus a stop later or get off a stop earlier
- Take a detour round the park
- Learn bowling or badminton
- Walk home from the pub or restaurant
- Sweep the floor
- Put on some music and dance
- Go for a country walk with friends

Walk, don't run!

One of the easiest ways to start being more active is to walk – you already know how to do it, you can wear anything you like, you probably have a pair of trainers or comfy shoes lurking in the wardrobe and it's free. Whether you choose somewhere close to home or further away is up to you – you just need to open the door and away you go.

Start by walking at your usual pace and when you feel a bit warmer, pick up the pace and walk briskly for a few minutes or for as long as you can. If you are walking in company you should be able to hold a conversation comfortably. Drop the pace towards the end of your walk to help your body get back to normal. Keep doing this every day or couple of days and you will soon be walking faster and feeling fitter.

Remember this is only a guide. Don't worry if you miss a few days or even a week – what is important is that you increase the effort bit by bit. Every day that you meet or exceed the target is a bonus.

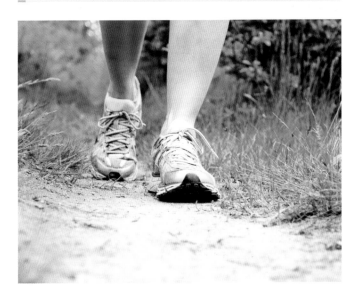

If you find it hard to get motivated to become more active, don't worry – you are not alone. In this day and age of busy lives and energy-saving devices, many people don't have the inclination to be particularly active or find they can't keep it up once they start. If this is the case with you, see if any of the motivational tips on pages 28 to 31 help. You might also want to use the activity log in the appendices, page 104. This will help you make a plan and also allows you to review your progress. Another option is to ask a friend or family member to support you – perhaps by agreeing to walk with you once a week, or by joining a class with you. Finally, remember that five minutes a day is better than nothing at all. Don't set your sights too high: start gently and work up.

A WORD OF CAUTION

If you are anxious about the health consequences of being more active, turn to page 61 and complete the health questionnaire. This is designed to highlight any health issues that might be affected by an increase in activity levels. If in doubt, it is always a good idea to talk through your plans with your GP. He or she will advise you on the level and kind of exercise that's right for you.

While activity and exercise will have a positive effect on both body and mind, worrying about it will add to your stress levels. If you genuinely think that it would increase your stress to start being more active, delay until you feel more able to cope. At the very lease, set aside five minutes a day to relax and be calm. Come back to the book when you are ready.

> YOU ARE WHAT YOU EAT

The food we eat affects how much energy we have and our health and wellbeing. There is lots of information about healthy eating available from a range of reputable and qualified sources, some of which are listed at the end of this book, so we won't go into too much detail here but it's worth looking at some of the basics.

Food for thought

Did you know that the chemicals in the brain that influence mood can be affected by the foods we eat? Many foods (especially processed) contain artificial chemicals, which can cause our body to react in different ways and affect our mood. Low levels of vitamins, minerals and essential fatty acids can also affect mental health: for instance, low levels of omega-3 oils (found in oily fish like sardines) have been linked to depression.

The charity Mind offers a wonderful guide to food and mood (see the 'find out more' section). Mind found that from a survey of 200 people, 88% reported that changing their diet for the better improved their feeling of wellbeing:

- 26% stated large improvements in mood swings
- 26% stated improvements in managing panic attacks and anxiety
- 24% stated improvements in their depression

Most of those surveyed said that cutting down on food 'stressors' and increasing the amount of food 'supporters' had a beneficial effect on their mood. This may be their subjective experience, but for whatever reason, it seems to be true that eating more healthily **does** have the potential to influence your mood.

Put some thought into your diet, think 'stressor' or 'supporter'. Here are some examples:

Stressor foods: include sugar, caffeine, alcohol, chocolate, processed food and food containing a large number of additives and saturated fats.

Supporter foods: include water, vegetables, fruit, nuts, fibre, seeds, wholegrain foods and oil-rich fish.

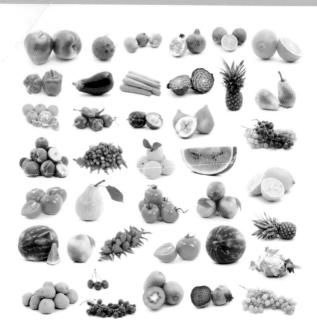

We all know that it's important to eat plenty of fresh fruit and vegetables – at least five portions a day. Some additional steps you can take to improve your diet are:

- Eating regularly and not skipping breakfast.
- Eating more complex carbohydrates such as brown rice or wholemeal bread.
- Eating less saturated fat.
- Eat less sugar and salt.
- Eating sufficient fibre.
- Balancing your calorie intake. Too few calories will slow down your metabolism and make you feel lethargic; too many calories will be stored as body fat and cause weight gain.
- Drinking more water. People often mix up feelings of hunger with thirst. If you are overweight, try taking a glass of water or fruit tea and see if you still feel hungry.
- Eating only when you feel hungry.

Many of us do eat healthy food – just too much. Stop eating earlier and wait for a few minutes to see if you still feel hungry – it actually takes about 20 minutes for our brain to register when we have had enough, so this gives you time to catch up!

> Use the 'food and mood' log on page 106 of the appendices to help you monitor the affects your diet is having on your mental wellbeing.

> ## FANCY A TIPPLE?

There are a significant number of physical health issues associated with drinking in excess of the recommended limits on a regular basis. These range from skin effects such as wrinkles, redness and dryness, to sleep and concentration problems.

Most people consider a drink in the evening to be a well-deserved reward for getting through the day and this is generally not a problem. However, alcohol is also a depressant so too much too often will have a psychological impact on our ability to cope with stress. Increased levels affect the chemistry of the brain, increasing the risk of depression by reducing the levels of the chemicals serotonin and noradrenaline that help us avoid depression. The long-term effects of alcohol can also create knock-on problems such as:

- Disturbed sleep or insomnia
- A constant low-level hangover that creates a cycle of waking up feeling ill, anxious, jittery and guilty
- Stress symptoms such as anxiety, guilt and sense of worthlessness
- Arguments with family or friends
- Work problems
- Memory loss
- Sexual problems such as impotence or low libido
- Osteoporosis

HOW MANY UNITS?

It's surprisingly easy to drink too much. Unfortunately, while the measure of an alcoholic drink has remained the same over the years – a pint or a half, a glass of wine, etc – the amount of alcohol contained in that measure has significantly increased. An average bottle of wine used to be 9% alcohol by volume (ABV) with 6 units in a bottle but now it is likely to be 13.5% or higher, containing at least 10 units. The same applies to beers and lagers – many are now higher than the standard 3.5% ABV twenty or so years ago. This means that many people are unknowingly drinking in excess of the recommended guidelines and increasing the risk factors for their health.

Recommended alcohol unit consumption		
Health risk	**Units of alcohol**	
	Women	**Men**
No significant health risks	2–3 units per day	3–4 units per day
Note: **It is advised that at least two days per week are alcohol-free**		
Increasing risk to health	3 or more units per day on a regular basis	4 or more units per day on a regular basis
A 'binge'	Drinking more than twice the recommended units in one 'session'	

(Adapted from: Department of Health public information leaflet 'Think about Drink' – www.drinkaware.co.uk)

A large glass of strong Australian red in the pub is about 3.4 units – over the daily recommendation for women! Drinking at home isn't any better as a bottle of wine probably has over 10 units and you may not notice how much you are drinking. A bottle of beer is nearly 2 units – two of them and you men are up to your daily allowance. Alcopops? There goes another 1.5 units.

Another issue is the growth of binge drinking in our culture. A binge is drinking more than twice the recommended daily amount in one 'session'. For women this would be 6 units in an evening (or two large glasses of wine in the pub) and for men it would be 8 units. People often binge drink when they're out with friends, so it can seem like a social activity rather than a harmful pastime.

If you're concerned about your drinking there is a wealth of support out there. Finding professional help, or joining a support group, can help you take control of this side of our life. See the 'find out more' section at the back of the book for more details.

> The pleasurable and relaxing effects of alcohol can be enjoyable, so if you are drinking within recommended limits it is unlikely to be harmful and need not be something to stress about!

> THE EVIL WEED

The negative consequences of cigarette smoking on health are well documented. Carbon monoxide and nicotine are the two chemicals in cigarettes that have the most impact on the heart. Carbon monoxide contributes to decreased oxygen being circulated around the body to the tissues. Nicotine stimulates the production of adrenaline, which increases heart rate and blood pressure, causing the heart to work harder. Smoking also damages the lining of the coronary arteries and contributes to atherosclerosis, a build-up of fatty tissue on the artery walls. The tar in cigarettes causes cancer.

Many people believe that smoking relaxes and de-stresses them, whereas it is more likely that the withdrawal symptoms have been alleviated by a cigarette, leading to a false sense of calmness.

Smoking is highly addictive and once started it isn't easy to quit. If you want to stop smoking, contact a local smoking cessation group via your GP surgery to receive advice and support to help you quit. (See the 'find out more' section for details of some information services.)

> **A MORNING JOLT**

That cup of coffee may perk you up in the morning but drinking too much over a long period can lead to a reliance on it to help you feel awake. Whether your choice is cola, coffee, tea or energy drinks makes no difference – they all create a false alertness that is followed by a slump in energy levels. Follow this with another 'shot' and then another and a cycle of highs and lows is created, which can affect how we sleep, our general health and energy levels. Caffeine also stimulates the nervous system, causing a faster heart rate and feelings of jitteriness.

One or two cups a day is fine and keeping this to the morning is better to avoid sleep problems at night. However, the effects of caffeine diminish substantially within three hours of drinking it so some people may be able to tolerate it later in the day. For most of us, switching to green tea, juice or water after lunch to keep hydrated and going for a brisk five-minute walk if we feel low in energy is enough to perk us up naturally.

Caffeine – how much are you drinking? A low to moderate intake of caffeine is 130–300mg per day.	
Product	**Caffeine (mg)**
Coffee	
Instant, weak (1 level tsp)	45
Instant, strong (1 heaped tsp)	90
Brewed, percolated, 20ml	100
Filtered, 200ml	140
Espresso (short black), 100ml	80
Cappuccino, 1 cup, 200ml	80
Tea	
Bag or brewed, weak, 200ml	20
Bag or brewed, strong, 200ml	70
Soft drinks	
Coke, 375ml	50
Pepsi, 375ml	38
Red Bull energy drink, 1 can, 250ml	80
Chocolate	
Dark, 50g	33
Milk, 50g	12

(Adapted from: *Choice Health Reader*, Jan/Feb 2001)

If you are consuming over 300mg a day it might be helpful to cut back, especially if you are struggling with sleep or are anxious. To reduce these negative symptoms try decaffeinated drinks, for example red bush tea, fruit teas or decaffeinated coffee. Alternatively, drink more water! It offers the body more hydration and is more refreshing and healthy.

> Habit is habit, and not to be flung out of the window, but coaxed downstairs a step at a time.
>
> **Mark Twain**

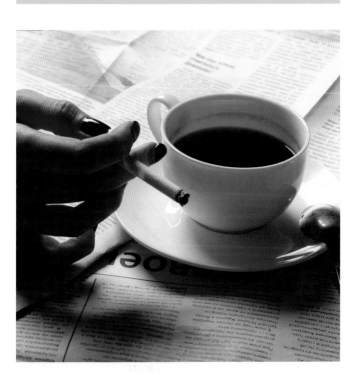

Habits are hard to break

So many of our traditional forms of relaxation – smoking, drinking, coffee – are actually stressors! They are also habits, and habits are hard to break…

This is true … but luckily it applies to good habits as well as bad ones!

Think about a positive habit that you have picked up recently – taking bags with you when you shop instead of endlessly collecting plastic ones, for example. This new habit was something you had to consciously remember to do at first and now it is probably something you do automatically. The same applies to stress-reducing habits – once you have practised them regularly over a period of time they will become automatic and you may even miss them when you don't do them.

Remember, there is nothing wrong with the odd lapse – just make sure it doesn't become a relapse.

Tips for replacing unhealthy habits with healthier habits:

- Eat a piece of fruit
- Drink a glass of water if you feel hungry – often you're actually just thirsty
- Go for a short walk when you get tired to refresh you
- Practise breathing exercises when you are stuck in traffic
- Meditate or relax for 5 minutes at the start and end of each day
- Perform some short desk relief exercises such as those on pages 70 to 72
- Go to an exercise session or join a regular walking group

Remember to give yourself a chance by starting gently. Don't quit smoking, booze and coffee all at once – you're quite likely to fail. Instead choose one, break it down, and take one step at a time:

Bad habit: skipping breakfast
End goal: balanced healthy breakfast
Start by: grabbing a healthy oat bar or a bottled smoothie on your way to work

> > **Super stress saviours**

Let's have a look at some ideas to help you reduce your stress levels. These are tricks that you can use on a regular basis as you go through life. Come back to them time and again and make them part of your daily coping mechanism.

> COPING WITH CATASTROPHISING

Ever woken up in the middle of the night and been unable to get back to sleep? Did you start to think about something and begin to worry, panic, think of the worst possible outcome and worry yourself into a state of stress, tension and fear? When you woke up (after finally falling asleep at 6 a.m.) did you wonder what on earth brought that on?

One of the side effects of stress is the tendency to 'catastrophise' even small things in a very negative way. In our minds, making a simple mistake at work becomes a very quick and rapid descent into being fired. We rarely think about a positive outcome.

It is hard to think positively when you are consumed with worry and negativity; however, it can help to create a positive-thinking coping strategy which will become a habit in the longer term. So, instead of using negative catastrophising, start to build a more positive thought process.

- If you wake up worried or stressed at night write down your concern or fear in a notebook and say firmly to yourself that you will deal with it in the morning. Things do look better in daylight, when we are able think more clearly.

- Start each day with a positive thought. Tell yourself that today is going to be OK, good, productive, sunny – whatever comes to mind. It may feel false at first but will soon become a habit.

- If you feel overwhelmed take a five-minute break, walk away, get some fresh air, breathe deeply, do a crossword, jump around, run up stairs, or do whatever distracts you for a few moments. You may find it easier when you return to the situation or task.

- Imagine a friend asking you for advice on whatever is bothering you – what would you tell them? Be honest: if you would tell them to grow up or stop whingeing or that it is not that bad, ask yourself *why* you are so worried about it.

- Take your biggest concern and imagine the worst possible outcome. How would you deal with it? What help or support is there from family, friends, the government? Often if we know we can cope with the worst scenario, the problem becomes less stressful. It may sound trivial but knowing that you are prepared for the worst really does help.

- Find a friend, counsellor or therapist who will listen with impartiality and not offer advice but who will let you talk yourself out. Often hearing our thoughts and fears spoken out loud enables us to rationalise them and find solutions, both temporary and permanent.

> **MEDITATION**

Every day, try to take time to sit quietly for five minutes or so and let unwanted or distracting thoughts pass by. Focus on your breathing and

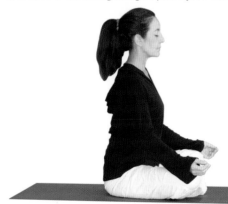

stillness. Any time will do and whenever you can – once the kids are in bed, just before you get up in the morning, or at lunchtime in the corner of a quiet park. Meditation is a great way of relaxing your mind and refreshing yourself.

A treat for your overworked mind

- Sit comfortably, back straight and supported, shoulders relaxed and arms resting on your lap
- Close your eyes
- Focus on breathing deeply and slowly for 10 counts
- Become aware of the activity of the mind and the speed of your thoughts
- Let the thoughts pass through the mind – let them go
- Focus on stillness
- Allow the mind to slow down
- Allow the mind to become quiet and silent
- Let go of other thoughts, acknowledge them, smile and release them
- Keep your focus on stillness
- Keep your focus on your breathing
- Allow the mind to rest
- Allow the mind to be free and peaceful

> ## SLEEP

Stress can disrupt the sleeping cycle – your normal sleeping patterns may be interrupted because your mind is racing with stressful or worrying thoughts. A healthy amount of sleep is essential, so it's important to develop healthy sleeping patterns.

Tips for developing healthy sleeping patterns:

- Make sure your bed and bedroom are at a comfortable temperature and not too noisy or light – you can get blackout blinds if your window is near a street light or if you are having difficulty sleeping on summer evenings when it stays light till late.

- If you can't sleep, the main thing is not to lie there getting frustrated but to get up and do something relaxing. Read or listen to quiet music. After a while you should feel sleepy enough to go back to bed.
- Keep to regular sleeping times – try to get to bed at the same time every night. Try to go to sleep and get up at the same time every day or as often as possible.
- Have a relaxing bath (maybe with candlelight) to help you to unwind before you go to bed. Water provides a comforting sensation for the body and soft lighting is restful for the eyes. Candles can be used as focus for meditation – you can watch the flame 'dance'.
- Make sure your mattress is comfy and supports you well. Change it every 10 years or so.
- Keep a notebook by your bed so that you can write down any thoughts that disrupt your sleeping patterns.
- Keep the bedroom for sleeping, rather than watching television or other activities.
- Try some relaxation or meditation before you go to bed.
- Listen to a relaxation tape or a positive-thinking tape when you go to bed to help you drift off to sleep.
- Don't exercise too close to when you go to bed – exercise earlier in the evening.
- Don't sleep during the day.
- Don't drink coffee or other stimulants before you go to bed.
- Don't drink alcohol before bedtime – you will sleep initially, but then wake up early.
- Don't smoke before bedtime.
- Don't eat your last meal close to bedtime.
- Don't use slimming tablets – many of these will keep you awake.

- Don't use drugs – many are stimulants.
- Don't go without sleep for a long time – stick to a routine.

> EXPRESS YOURSELF

Rather than bottling up the things you think or feel, write them down in a journal or in the form of a letter. If you are artistic (and even of you aren't) you can draw a picture or use clay or even driftwood to make a sculpture. Feelings are better out than in and they need an outlet. Sometimes it is not the right time to express specific thoughts to a person; writing the thoughts in a letter will enable you to release them. It may make you cry at first and/or it may trigger the feeling that 'I am bad to think these thoughts' – let go of the guilt and let go of the thoughts. Creativity offers an outlet that is safe.

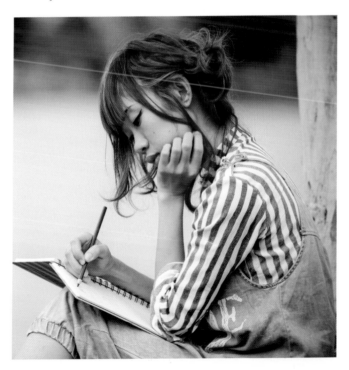

> When I feel angry at someone, I write an angry letter (which I don't send) or I scribble a picture or write words – it gets the feelings out. Then when I feel better, I can decide if I want to be assertive and express my feelings in a way that is helpful to the relationship I have with the person.
>
> Or, when I am feeling low and I don't understand it, I write a poem, or what I call a 'word soup'. This shows me on paper what I am feeling, and as a visual person, it helps me to understand myself.
>
> **Sue, aged 25**

> ASSERT YOURSELF

One of the biggest causes of stress for many people is being over-whelmed with things to do. Often this comes from being unable or unwilling to say no, sometimes as a way of gaining or keeping approval from others and not from a genuine desire to be helpful. The problem is that if you keep saying yes, people may not realise that they are asking too much, so part of learning to manage stress is learning that saying no is important too. You may find that you are very good at saying no in one area of your life and are unable to say no in others.

PRACTISE BEING MORE ASSERTIVE

Becoming more assertive takes time – you need to believe what you are saying in order to appear in control and this is not easy for some. The following steps are useful to help you take back control of your time:

- Decide want you want
- State what you want clearly and specifically
- Use positive and confident body language
- Use 'I' statements – I feel, I think (rather than 'you should' or 'you make me')
- Listen to the other person

- Stay focused
- Aim for a win–win situation
- Manage and respect your feelings

Know your rights ... I have the right to:	
Ask for what I want	Not know about something
Say: 'No'	Choose whether to get involved with the problems of another
Have and express my own opinions, feelings and thoughts	Make mistakes
Make my own decisions and manage the consequences	Say: 'I don't understand'
Change my mind	Be treated with respect
Have time for myself	Act assertively
Be successful	Choose not to assert myself

(Adapted from: Bayne et al. (1998:7), *The Counsellors Handbook*)

> ### TICK TOCK

Modern life is hectic – long working hours, commuting, family commitments and the need to 'have it all' can make us feel like we're running just to keep up. To manage our precious time so that we have some for ourselves, we need to:

- Identify what our priorities are and share our time equally among these
- Recognise the less important, time-wasting activities
- Not take on more than we can handle (and learn to say 'No!')
- Delegate tasks or ask for help and support if we need it
- Not forget to make time for ourselves and for activities we enjoy that will help to manage stress.

Top tips for managing your time

- **Write a list:** Whether it's at work or at home, make a list of things that need to get done, with the most urgent or important at the top. Tackle the things that you hate doing first so that they get done and don't get overlooked or carried over onto the list for the next day. For example do the filing before you plan your business trip. At home do the housework before you do the gardening.
- **Get 'chunky':** Break large or unpleasant tasks into smaller chunks to make them easier to tackle. For example, if you don't like doing your accounts start by getting all your receipts together. Then put them in date order and input them onto a spreadsheet. Next tackle your income and so on. It make take you a few days but, as each chunk is shorter than the whole task, it will be much less stressful to do.
- **Remove interruptions:** Use answer-phones, 'do not disturb' signs on the office door and check your emails at set times to avoid being distracted. Set your work phone to switch off at 8pm and back on at 8am so you are not tempted to look at it or carry on working during your home time.
- **Stick to a routine:** Plan your time and you'll be amazed at how much more you can get done – leaving you more 'me' time! Use a diary to plan a routine to get things done (including exercise) and try to stick to it as much as possible.
- **Pace yourself:** Remember to take regular breaks, and it will make your working time more focused and effective. Save the activities that you love doing for your tired moments as these will lift your mood.
- **Advance meal planning:** Cook more than you need and freeze portions, and book supermarket shops online once a week to save on the supermarket scramble
- **Pay other people:** If you can afford to, employ a cleaner or gardener or get a babysitter in to give you some free time.
- **Me, me, me**: If you never make time in your diary for yourself, then no wonder you feel stressed. Making time for yourself and booking time in your diary for things that you want to do are essential for maintaining a healthy life balance.

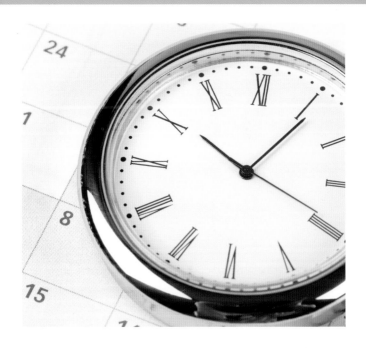

Whatever you are doing, whether it is work, family time, exercise or a hobby, try to focus only on that particular thing. Don't let thoughts of your 'to-do' list interrupt the moment.

> LAUGHTER IS THE BEST MEDICINE

If you feel miserable or stressed try smiling for a while – it reduces the negative tension around the face and relaxes the facial muscles and often it brings about a more positive feeling. If you have forgotten how to smile, start adding smiles to your daily routine. Fake it till you make it!

Laughter offers an incredible release for stress but so many of us get out of the habit of it. Find something that gives you a good belly laugh. If you have forgotten how to laugh, rent some comedy movies and watch them all until you become infected with laughter.

Oh, and laughter is a very good workout for the tummy muscles so double the reason to giggle!

Apparently children laugh over 300 times a day and adults only manage a measly 15 times. While adults tend to laugh at something specific, children laugh unconditionally – just for the fun of it!

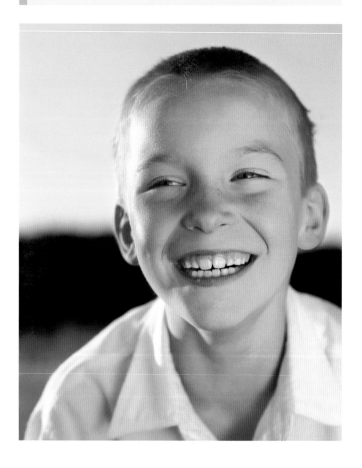

Creature comforts

Make regular time for some creature comforts and things that make you feel good. This is your 'you' time and it's an important part of staying relaxed and combating stress. Here are a few ideas of ways to treat yourself and unwind in body and mind:

- Hot, fragrant bubble-bath in candlelight with soft music
- Writing a letter to a friend
- Having a massage
- Curling up on the sofa with a video
- Sofa and a face pack
- Manicure and pedicure
- Horse riding in the countryside
- Day at a health spa
- Watching a feel-good film
- Dancing to a piece of music
- Daydreaming
- Gardening
- Cuddling up with my teddy and letting myself feel sorry for myself
- Going for a walk with my partner
- Listening to music on my own
- Sleeping
- Drawing pictures
- Booking a short break or holiday, so I have something to look forward to
- Drinking a cup of hot chocolate
- Driving to a place with great scenic views – with no cars, no people, no phones
- Walking my dog, taking a flask of tea and snacks
- Going for a run
- Cooking myself a special, healthy and nourishing meal
- Baking a cake
- Lighting a fire
- Doing some knitting
- Watching a match on TV with a beer or two

Note: Thanks to all the wonderful people who contributed their personal creature comforts to develop this list.

> ## FEEL THE FEAR AND DO IT ANYWAY

Is there something that you would really like to do but are afraid of trying, in case you fail or are no good at it?

Managing fear plays an important role in managing stress. Fear is an emotion that we all experience whenever we do something that moves us out of our comfort zone. The key is how we manage the fear and whether we allow it to rule us.

One way of managing fear is to set life targets that extend our personal comfort zone. Each time we achieve a target, our comfort zone expands and we feel good. And even if we don't always achieve the target, we can congratulate ourselves on the fact that we had a go!

If fear is an issue for you, a brilliant book to read is *Feel the Fear and Do It Anyway* by Susan Jeffers. This is a really motivational and inspirational book about how to manage fear and the change process.

> ## RELAXATION

Relaxing for five minutes every day can be incredibly positive. It doesn't take long to collect yourself, rest and feel better.

It's not always easy to relax instantly though, especially as we get older. It takes practise – and here are some tips to help you.

1. Actively contracting and then relaxing each of your muscles can help release tension and create a relaxed feeling. You may find it hard to be still initially, but if you keep practicing, it will become much easier and more natural and you will feel better.
2. Buy a relaxation audio book or download it onto your MP3 player. You can even read and record the relaxation script in the appendices at the back of the book (see page 108), and play it to yourself whenever you need help relaxing.
3. Use the Benson method of relaxation, which uses breathing and repetition to help calm and relax you.

Dr Herbert Benson developed his own method of relaxation to treat patients with high blood pressure. He suggested that individuals sit still and quietly focus on their breathing and, on every outward breath, say out loud the word 'one'.

The technique can be adapted in the following ways:

- The word 'one' can be replaced by other words that you find more natural, such as 'calm', 'peace', 'love', 'still', 'silent' or 'relax', or even a mantra or chant, such as 'om'.
- The technique can be used in everyday activities, for example when queuing at a supermarket, travelling on the train, sitting at an office desk or walking.
- It can be used while sitting, standing or lying.

The five-minute version

- Sit quietly with an open, relaxed body posture
- Focus on your breathing
- As you breathe out, focus on a desired word or mantra
- The word chosen can be spoken out loud or quietly within
- Practise this for about five minutes, just allowing the body to relax

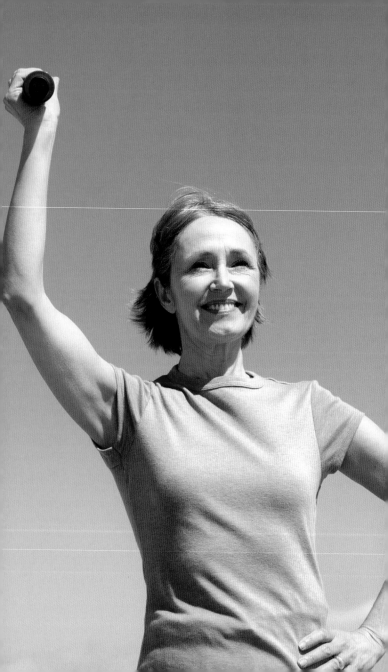

part

3

the exercises

Our body is designed to move: the skeleton is made up of many joints that enable us to move in lots of different directions, and muscles that grow stronger with use. If we don't use the body, we lose some of the potential to move it and become stiff and immobile. This creates physical tension and a build-up of stress, and can contribute to some of the modern-day diseases that are linked to inactivity, such as obesity, arthritis, osteoporosis, diabetes, high blood pressure and coronary heart disease.

Some of the physical benefits of exercise

- Increases the strength of our heart
- Improves the circulation of blood and oxygen around the body
- Improves the rate at which we breathe
- Improves the tone and strength of our muscles
- Improves the strength of our bones
- Lowers our blood cholesterol levels
- Lowers our blood pressure
- Improves our mood
- Provides an outlet for tension and stress
- Reduces the risk of depression
- Burns calories and helps us to manage our weight

>> Exercise and stress

As you will have noticed from reading the first part of this book, stress can have long-term effects on the body and mind. Building activity into everyday life can help to manage stress in the following ways:

- **Helps use the fight or flight response in the right way**. When we are active we use up the nervous energy that builds up when we are stressed. Exercise uses the fight and flight energy in the way it was intended: we may not be fighting or fleeing, but we are channelling the energy rather than letting it build up to create tension and disharmony in our body.

- **Release of chemicals**. Activity increases the levels of feel-good chemicals, including endorphins, in our system. These create a pleasant 'high', which makes us feel better, and also include serotonin and noradrenaline, which are found in lower levels in people with depression and anxiety.

- **Warm up**. Exercise and activity raise our body temperature and it is known that when our bodies are warmer, muscle tension reduces.

- **Feel better**. People tend to feel better when their health is good. Compare how you feel when you have a cold with how you feel on a good day. Which would you prefer?

- **Improved sleep patterns**. It is hard to feel good when sleep patterns are disturbed for any length of time. Being active helps to create a pleasant physical tiredness and improve the length and quality of sleep. As the old saying goes: 'It will all seem better after a good night's sleep.'

- **Greater belief in ourselves and our ability and potential**. Exercise can help to improve our confidence. It provides a sense of achievement and pride that goes with successful completion of a task or chore. Completing an activity session means that there is at least one thing 'done and dusted today'.

- **A better body image**. Regular activity helps to maintain a healthy weight and improve our muscle tone and posture. The effect of this is being more comfortable with our body, which is in itself a mind-boosting feeling. It is also suggested that regular exercisers 'see' a better body in the mirror than those who are inactive, even when there are no real physical differences.

- **Distraction**. During exercise or activity it is easy to forget troubles or problems. Many people find that distracting themselves from a problem helps them to find a solution more easily or just gives some breathing space for the mind. If we stop thinking about the stressor, our stress response diminishes.

- **Time out/me time**. Taking time out from the stress and workload of the day can provide a real break and when this includes some activity it can revitalise and refresh the mind and body and help us cope with what comes our way.

- **Increased resistance to stress**. Being active appears to make us more resistant to stress, as regular exercisers show lower levels of stress or anxiety when in a stressful situation than people who are not active.

If someone invented a pill that did all of this, the makers would be overwhelmed with demand – and yet we can have it all just by becoming more active. So let's start!

> > The starting point

This part of the book contains different exercise plans that you can do at home or outdoors if you prefer, along with some suggestions for other types of exercise. The exercises can be done for 5 minutes, 30 minutes or anything that works for you, so you can adapt them as you wish. These are ideal for exercising in private, but don't forget that there are other options.

Classes at leisure centres, gyms or studios cater for all tastes, ages and levels of fitness. You don't have to do kick-boxing or intense aerobics: there are Pilates or yoga classes where students are encouraged to go at their own pace, or you could try aqua aerobics – a fun and gentle form of exercise. Or why not join a dancing class? The added bonus is that you can take a breather when you need to.

Don't be put off by the idea that everyone at the gym or in a class is really fit either. Most classes will be full of red-faced, out-of-breath people having a good time. The best attitude is to give it your best shot and forget about appearances. If you're in any doubt that the class is right for you, try to get in touch with the instructor and have a talk with them beforehand. They will let you know what level of fitness is required, and help you make a choice that suits you.

>> Safety first

Before going any further, you need to run through a few questions designed to highlight any health problems that might affect your ability to exercise. Complete the questionnaire on page 61. Have you answered 'yes' to any of the questions? If so, you should go and speak to your doctor before getting more active or taking exercise. They will be able to advise you on exercising at a level that is safe for you.

There are plenty of options for people of any age with health conditions or a low level of fitness, so don't be downhearted. From exercise classes designed specifically for older people to gentle chair-based exercises to swimming, there will be something for you. The main thing is that you approach any new exercise with an understanding of your physical condition and limitations – that way you can exercise at a level that's safe and rewarding for you.

> I have suffered from a bad back for much of my adult life. The pain contributed to my stress and prevented me from taking exercise.
> Then my doctor suggested Pilates. Not only do my weekly classes relax me, but they have strengthened my stomach muscles and that have done wonders for my back!

Richard, aged 43

Health questionnaire		
Are you fit to get physical?	yes	no
1 Has your doctor ever said you have a heart or vascular condition and/or that you should only do activity recommended or supervised by a doctor?		
2 Do you feel any pain in your chest when you do physical activity?		
3 In the past month have you had chest pain when you were not doing physical activity?		
4 Do you lose your balance because of dizziness or other reasons or do you ever lose consciousness?		
5 Do you have a bone or joint problem that is affected by or could be made worse by physical activity?		
6 Is your doctor currently prescribing medication for any condition?		
7 Are you over 69 years of age and not used to physical activity?		
8 Do you know of any reason why you should not take part in physical activity?		
9 Are you pregnant now or have you been pregnant in the last six months?		
10 Have you been diagnosed with a medical condition in the last two months?		
11 Are you significantly overweight?		

If you have answered yes to any of the questions please discuss the answers with your doctor who will advise you on whether it is the right time to become more active.

If you answered no to all of them, you are ready to up your exercise and activity levels.

Before you start exercising, you need to make sure you follow some safety guidance first:

- When you are exercising wear loose-fitting, comfortable clothing and a supportive, comfortable pair of trainers.

- If you are exercising outdoors, make sure you wear appropriate clothing and take precautions to keep warm or protect yourself against the environment (use sunscreen in summer).

- For personal safety, always take a mobile phone with you and make sure you tell someone where you are going.

- If you feel thirsty, sip water throughout, but avoid taking long drinks.

- If you have eaten a heavy meal, wait two hours before exercising.

- If you want to exercise but feel hungry, have a light snack like a banana or a piece of toast. It is useful to have a small snack immediately after any activity to replace the nutrients you need to replenish your energy stores.

- Do what feels comfortable. If anything feels uncomfortable, don't do it. It may not be right for your body.

- Only exercise when you feel well and healthy. Do not exercise if you have a cold or flu or if you are excessively tired.

- Make sure there is enough space around you. Move any chairs, tables or bags out of the way.

- Check your posture before you start (see page 64).

- Breathe naturally at all times and never hold your breath.

- Always complete the warm-up before you move on to the other exercises.

- Always stretch at the end of your routine.

- Do not force yourself to work too hard or complete a difficult movement or exercise.

> > How often and hard should I exercise?

When you are taking part in physical activity and exercise, it is essential to monitor how hard you are working, not just how long you are working for. The scale shown in the table below provides a useful way for you to check that you are working at the right level. It can help you to recognise how much energy you are putting in to the activity/exercise.

Working at the right level		
Number rating	How it feels for you?	
1	Very light	I could keep this going all day
2	Light	I feel a little warmer
3	Moderate	I can feel my heart beating a bit faster and I am breathing heavier
4	Somewhat hard	This feels harder but I am still comfortable
5	Getting harder	I am really feeling it now but not too bad
6	Hard	Ooh, this is barely comfortable
7	Harder	Uncomfortable now, I can't do this for long
8	Very hard	Very uncomfortable and I cannot keep going
9	Very, very hard	I need to stop, this feels awful
10	Maximum	I'm about to collapse

Aim to work at a level between 3 and 4 when performing activities

Remember that you can build an increase in physical activity into your life very easily, whether you're walking to work or doing some simple exercises. But how much should you do? Well, all exercise is good for you. Even five minutes extra a day can improve your health over time. Ideally though, you should exercise for half an hour five times a day. See the table on page 64 for more information.

Targets to work towards	
Frequency	Aim to be active on at least 5 days of the week. You can start with 1 day a week at first and build up.
Intensity	When you are moving, you need to work at a level where you feel a little breathless but comfortable. This will be different for each person: some people may find walking up the stairs easy and some may find it hard work.
Time	Being active for 30 minutes each day is ideal. You can break this down into shorter intervals throughout the day: try a short 10-minute walk, and repeat it 3 times during the day.
Type	Choose any activity that fits well into your daily lifestyle, that you like doing and that you know you have the potential to keep up.

>> **Posture and breathing**

It's all too easy to spend time slumped at your desk, huddled in the train or car as you commute, or walking with shoulders stooped and head down. But poor posture of this sort can lead to a range of different physical problems, from repetitive strain injury to back ache. It can also have an impact on your mood, it affects how people percieve you, and can stop you breathing fully and deeply.

Correcting poor posture can take time. You have to keep reminding yourself to sit or stand properly, which can be difficult if you're feeling tired or demoralised. But keep at it – very soon it will become second nature to you. You can do it anytime you remember – waiting for the kettle to boil, standing in queues, sitting in traffic, etc.

If you are exercising, it's extremely important to start from a position of good posture. Practise by looking in the mirror as you go through the steps below. You could even ask a friend or colleague to examine your posture, and you could do the same for them in return.

> ## STEPS TO CORRECT STANDING POSTURE

- Stand with your feet parallel and hip-width apart

- Distribute your weight between heel bone, big toe and little toe

- Spread your toes, aligning second toe with knee and hip

- Find a neutral pelvic position – it should not be tipped forwards or backwards

- Lengthen your torso and neck

- Tighten your deeper abdominal (tummy) muscles by visualising that you are zipping up a tight pair of trousers

- Look forwards, keeping your chin parallel to the floor

- Keeping your shoulders relaxed, slide your shoulder blades down towards your buttocks

- Keep your hands by the sides of your body, palms facing forwards

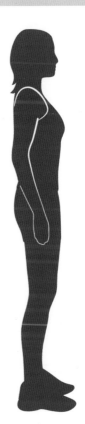

Instant stress relief

Are you at home, in a bookshop or sitting at your desk at work? Stop what you are doing right now and open your posture! Notice how much better it feels to lengthen your spine and lift up from your torso, not just physically but mentally too.

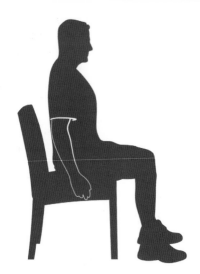

> **STEPS TO CORRECT SEATED POSTURE**
- Sit on the front third of the chair
- Place your feet parallel and hip-width apart
- Distribute your weight evenly between heel bone, big toe and little toe and spread your toes
- Sit upright and lengthen your spine
- Lift out of your sitting bones to find a neutral pelvic position (minimal forward or backward tilt of pelvis)
- Lengthen your torso and neck
- Tighten your abdominals
- Look forwards, keeping your chin parallel to the floor
- Keeping your shoulders relaxed, slide your shoulder blades down
- Place your hands by the sides of the chair, palms facing forwards

> **BREATHING**

Correct breathing enables us to take more oxygen into the lungs. Abdominal breathing allows the breath to move into deeper areas of the lungs. Since many of us breathe very shallowly most of the time we are missing out on the positive effects of good breathing practise.

Breathing correctly can help to improve the posture of the upper spine, keep the spine more mobile and prevent tension building up. Correct breathing can stop us from becoming too stressed in the first place. If we focus on breathing correctly and deeply, our breathing rate slows down and other body systems also relax – the heart rate can slow down slightly and the muscles relax. All in all, it is extremely good for you!

When exercising, many people accidentally hold their breath. It's important to use your breathing to your advantage, breathing deeply and easily through your exercises. You can also use the breath to help you by breathing out on the effort – the lifting phase of the movement – and in on the lowering phase of the exercise. Don't worry if this sounds complicated: it will come naturally with practise.

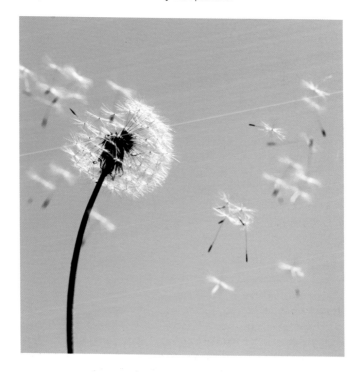

Breathing exercise

- Start by finding a relaxed position, seated, lying or standing

- Focus on the depth, speed and feeling of your breathing

- Close your eyes or focus on a specific spot looking forwards or slightly downwards (make sure your posture position doesn't change)

- Take the breath slightly deeper into the lower rib cage (most people take very shallow breaths into the upper chest area)

- Keep the breath soft, smooth and rhythmical

- Find a natural breathing pace and power

- Let the breath become effortless and allow it to flow freely

- Notice your abdomen rise and fall

- Allow your lower rib cage to expand sideways (you can place your hands around the ribs if it helps)

- Allow a few minutes just to focus on the breathing and stillness

>> Exercise programmes

It's time to get started. There are lots of different kinds of exercises illustrated in this section. From chair-based exercises suitable for the workplace (see page 70) to the high-energy cardiovascular workout on page 84, you should be able to pick and mix a routine that suits your mood.

If you are not used to exercise, select **one** of the routines to start with – ideally the warm-up routine – and practise a couple of exercises at first. Then gradually add in more when you feel ready for a longer workout. You can mix and match exercises from the different routines to design your own workout. Perhaps you want to do cardio one day and stretching the next? Whatever you do, keep your legs moving all the time using marching on the spot if you can, and substitute this for any exercises you find too challenging.

It's important that you work at a pace and level that suit you. Listen to your body and adjust your workout accordingly. It's far better to start with a few easy exercises that you find comfortable and do them well and often, than try to do everything at once. If you're feeling low or very busy or stressed, just stick to a few simple exercises – it won't be too daunting and will make you feel much better.

Always remember to warm up first, and cool down with stretches at the end. You should aim to begin gently, work a little harder in the middle of your routine and then gradually work down.

Note: All routines can vary in length, depending on how many repetitions of each exercise you do, and how many exercises you choose to perform. A good starting point is 5 to 10 minutes of the mobility and warming routine – then add in other exercises as you see fit.

> I was unhappy at work. My job was stressful and I never took a proper break. I could feel that my body was being affected, as well as my mind. So I set myself a target: to take a five-minute break in the morning and practise a short desk-relief routine.
>
> Doing the desk-relief exercises and the breathing focus allowed me to switch off for five minutes and focus on me. It helped because I knew I was doing something good for my body and mind. My posture improved and so did my breathing, and I felt much happier when tackling problems for the rest of the day.
>
> **David, 42**

DESK-RELIEF EXERCISES

Many of us spend a great deal of time sitting at a desk or in a chair. This can contribute to stiffness and tension. This section describes a simple routine of six exercises that can be practised anytime, anywhere, to help you feel more relaxed and flexible.

For all seated exercises start from a position of good posture. You should have a straight back with your tummy tucked in, you neck long, shoulders relaxed and your feet hip-width apart.

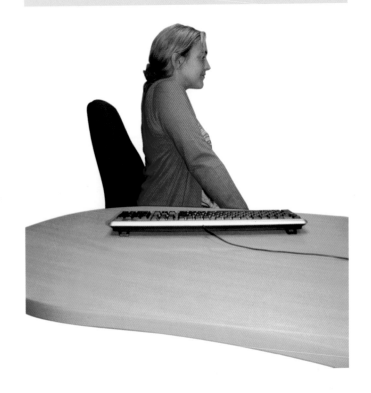

1. SHOULDER ROLLS

1 Maintain an upright posture and engage your abdominals
2 Roll your shoulders forwards, upwards and then backwards and down
3 Perform 8–12 repetitions

2. SIDE BENDS

1 Lift your torso and bend to one side in a controlled manner
2 Return to the central position
3 Lift and bend to the other side in a controlled manner
4 Return to the central position
5 Only bend as far over as is comfortable
6 Visualise your body as being placed between two panes of glass as you bend
7 Perform 8–12 repetitions

3. SIDE TWISTS

1 Hold your arms comfortably in front of you at shoulder level, with the elbows slightly bent
2 Twist around to one side
3 Come gently back to the centre
4 Then twist to the other side
5 Keep your hips facing forwards
6 Keep your chest lifted and shoulders relaxed and down
7 Perform 8–12 repetitions

4. CHAIR MARCHING

1 Sit upright with your feet hip-width apart, knees bent and abdominals engaged
2 March your legs gently, maintaining an upright posture
3 Keep this going for 1 minute, have a rest then repeat

5. HEEL DIGS

1 Dig alternate heels to the floor in front of your body, maintaining an upright posture

2 Keep this going for 1 minute, have a rest then repeat

6. CHEST STRETCH

1 Take your hands behind you and hold the back of your chair

2 Lean forwards slightly until a mild tension is felt at the front of the chest

3 Keep your elbows slightly bent

4 Squeeze your shoulder blades together and lift your chest to increase the stretch

5 Hold the stretch for 8–12 seconds

Note: Your hands can also be placed on your buttocks or clasped together behind your back – whichever is most comfortable.

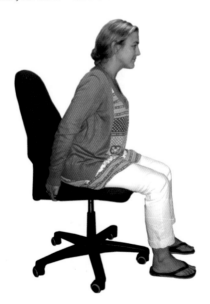

THE WARM-UP
These standing exercises are designed to loosen the joints and give a better range of movement. They prevent the body becoming stiff and immobile and also help to improve posture. Some of the movements will get the muscles warm and increase the heart rate and may activate the release of endorphins – the feel-good hormones. Remember to start from a good posture position with your back straight and your tummy tucked in, and breathe naturally throughout.

1. SHOULDER ROLLS

❶ Gently roll your shoulders forwards, then up and backwards and finally downwards

❷ As you lower your shoulders, feel your shoulder blades slide down towards your buttocks

❸ Perform 8–12 repetitions

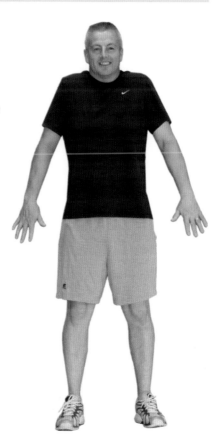

2. SIDE BENDS

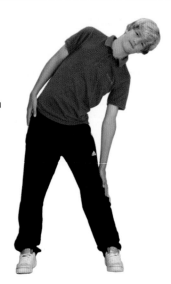

1 Bend directly to the side in a controlled manner and return to the central position
2 Bend directly to the other side in a controlled manner and return to the central position
3 Visualise your body as being placed between two panes of glass and bend only as far over as is comfortable
4 Keep your hips facing forwards and the movement controlled
5 Keep your body lifted between the hips and the ribs
6 Perform 8–16 repetitions on each side (alternating)

3. SIDE TWISTS

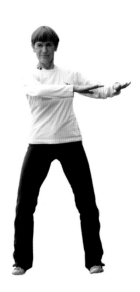

1 Start with your feet shoulder width and a half apart
2 Hold out your arms at shoulder level, with your elbows slightly bent or place your hands on hips
3 Twist around to one side, back to the centre and then twist to the other side
4 Twist only as far around as is comfortable
5 Keep your hips and knees facing forwards
6 Perform 8–16 repetitions on each side (alternating)

4. LEG CURLS

① Start with your feet hip-width apart
② Step out to the right and transfer your weight over to your right leg, kicking your left heel towards the buttocks
③ Step your left leg down and transfer your weight onto this leg, kicking your right heel to the buttocks
④ Take a large but comfortable stride of the legs
⑤ Keep your hips facing forwards and avoid hollowing the lower back by tightening your abdominal muscles
⑥ Ensure that your knee joint remains unlocked when landing
⑦ Keep the movement controlled, smooth and not jerky
⑧ Perform 8–16 repetitions on each side (alternating)

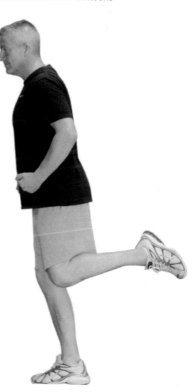

5. HEEL AND TOE

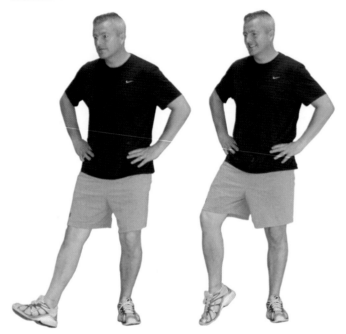

① Start with your feet hip-width apart and take your weight onto one leg
② Dig the heel of your free foot towards the floor and then point the toe towards the floor
③ Keep your weight-bearing leg soft, your hips facing forwards and the movement controlled
④ Aim for the heel and toe to land in the same place
⑤ Repeat on the other leg
⑥ Perform 8–16 repetitions on each side (alternating)

6. KNEE LIFTS

1 Start with your feet shoulder width and a half apart
2 Start raising alternate knees in front of your body
3 Take a comfortable stride of the legs
4 Keep your hips facing forwards
5 Lift your leg only to a height where an upright spine alignment can be maintained
6 Keep your chest lifted and do not allow your body to bend forwards as your leg lifts
7 Perform for 1–2 minutes

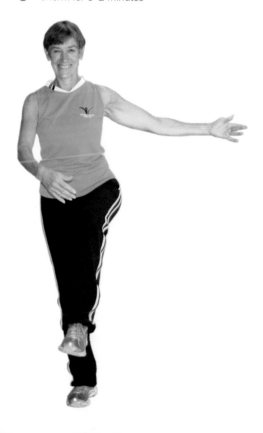

7. MARCHING/WALKING

1 Start with your feet hip-width apart

2 Maintain an upright posture and engage your abdominals

3 Start marching or walking on the spot

4 Land your feet lightly

5 Keep your knees unlocked

6 You can play music and perform this movement for longer and/or combine it with some of the other mobility movements

7 You can also travel this movement forwards and backwards or around the room

8 Perform for 2–4 minutes

Note: Marching can be used as a warm-up in its own right. It will raise your heart rate and warm your muscles. It can also be used between exercises as well as between repetitions of exercises as you build up strength and stamina.

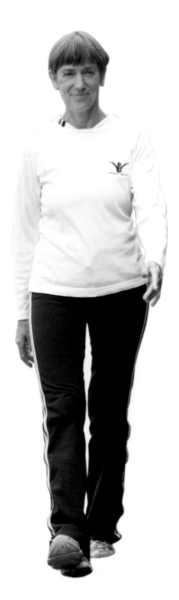

STRETCH IT OUT!

These exercises reduce any tightness and can lengthen the muscles. They improve the efficiency of our movements and can help to make daily tasks easier. Stretching also assists with relaxation and can improve posture. It's a good idea to stretch after a warm-up and before moving on to other exercises. Stretching is also an important part of the warm down. Only stretch as far as is comfortable and remember to hold a stretch – don't bounce.

1. HAMSTRING STRETCH

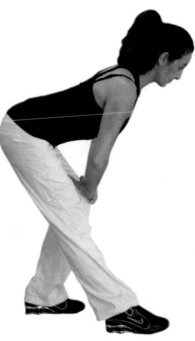

1 Step one leg forwards – a shoulder-width stride

2 Bend the knee of your back leg and place your hands at the top of your thigh of the bent knee

3 Bend forwards from the hips, supporting your weight with your hand on the bent knee

4 Stop when a mild tension is felt at the back of the thigh of the straight leg

5 Keep the knee of your straight leg fully extended, but not locked out

6 Keep your spine long and your chest lifted

7 Hold the stretch for 10–15 seconds

8 Repeat on the other leg

2. QUADRICEP STRETCH

❶ Balance on one leg – use a wall or chair to support you

❷ Raise the opposite foot towards your buttocks until a mild tension is felt at the front of the thigh

❸ Use your hand to hold the leg in place

❹ Keep your supporting knee joint unlocked

❺ Make sure your heel lifts towards the centre of your body, not to the side

❻ Tilt your pelvis slightly forwards

❼ Keep both knee joints in line with each other

❽ Hold the stretch for 10–15 seconds

❾ Repeat on the other leg

3. CALF STRETCH

❶ Step your right leg backwards as far as possible and with the heel of this back foot on the floor

❷ Keep your front knee bent but do not let your knee roll inwards

❸ Keep your hips facing forwards

❹ Visualise a straight line running from your ear to the ankle of your extended leg

❺ Use a wall or chair to support you

❻ Hold the stretch for 10–15 seconds

❼ Repeat on the other leg

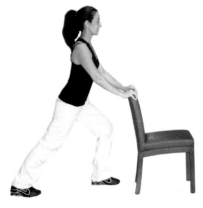

4. ADDUCTOR STRETCH

1 Lunge to the side, taking your body weight onto the bent leg
2 Keep your other leg extended, knee straight but not locked
3 Keep the hips facing forwards and avoid hollowing the lower back
4 Use a wall for support if you need to
5 Hold the stretch for 10–15 seconds
6 Repeat on the other leg

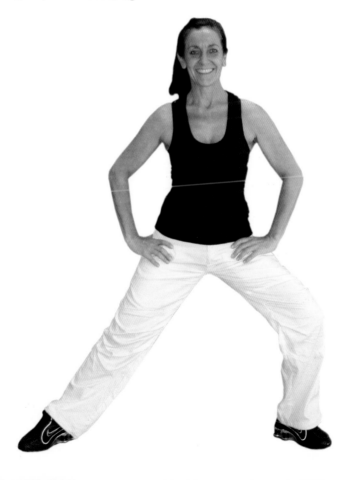

5. OBLIQUE STRETCH

1 Start with your feet shoulder width and a half apart

2 Place one hand on your hip to support your body weight

3 Raise your other arm up and bend over slightly to the side

4 Keep the knee joint of both legs slightly bent

5 Emphasise lifting your body upwards rather than leaning too far over to the side

6 Stretch only to a point where a mild tension is felt at the side of your trunk

7 Keep your body weight equally divided between your legs and avoid pushing your hip out to the side

8 When bending to the side, move your body in a straight line and without leaning forwards or backwards

9 Hold the stretch for 10–15 seconds

10 Repeat on the other side

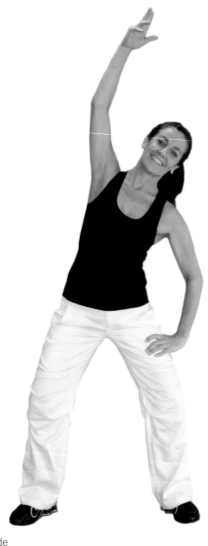

6. TRICEP STRETCH

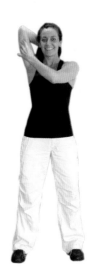

❶ Start with your feet shoulder width and a half apart
❷ Place one hand over your head on the centre of your back
❸ Use your other arm to ease the arm further down
❹ Hold the position with your knees slightly bent
❺ Stretch only to a point where a mild tension is felt at the back of your upper arm
❻ Hold the stretch for 10–15 seconds
❼ Repeat on the other arm

7. CHEST STRETCH

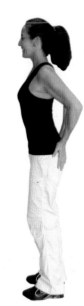

❶ Start with your feet shoulder width and a half apart
❷ Take your hands backwards until a mild tension is felt at the front of your chest – your hands can be placed on your buttocks or clasped together behind your back, whichever is most comfortable
❸ Keep your knees unlocked
❹ Keep your elbows slightly bent
❺ Slide your shoulder blades down and lift your chest to increase the stretch
❻ Hold the stretch for 10–15 seconds

CARDIO
This cardiovascular routine is designed to make our heart and circulatory system stronger. It will also contribute to the release of endorphins providing the feel-good factor, which can last for a long time after the initial activity has ended. It's important to perform five minutes of mobility and warming exercises first and ideally some stretches too, and to stretch at the end. Start gently, work harder in the middle then ease up. Take care doing impact exercises like jogging if you have joint problems, and always go at your own speed.

1. MARCH OR JOG ON THE SPOT
Jogging and marching on the spot can help keep you warm between exercises. They are also great cardiovascular activities in their own right. Depending on your level of fitness, use marching or jogging for a few minutes on their own, to keep you warm between exercises, or as a break between repetitions of the same exercise.

2. SQUATS WITH ARM CIRCLES
❶ Start with your feet two hip-widths apart, so that when you bend your knees they stay in line with your toes
❷ Bend your knees to a 90-degree angle
❸ Straighten them again without locking your knees
❹ Add a circling movement of your arms in front of your body to raise the intensity
❺ Start with 30 seconds and then march for 30 seconds

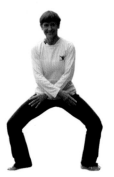 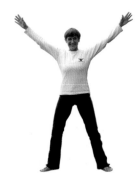

3. LUNGES

1. Maintain an upright posture and engage your abdominals
2. Lunge to the side, keeping your hips facing forwards
3. Step back and repeat
4. Start with 30 seconds and then go back to marching or jogging for 30 seconds

Note: you can add some forward or backward lunges to vary your routine

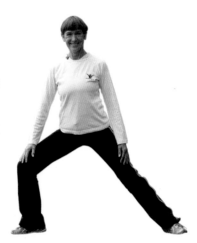

4. LEG KICKS

1. Kick alternate legs out in front of your body
2. You can add a hop at the same time if it feels comfortable
3. Keep your hopping knee joint unlocked and make sure your heel goes down
4. Take care not to lock the knee of your kicking leg
5. Start with 30 seconds, then march for 30 seconds to reduce the impact on the joints

Note: Gradually build up the number of cycles of kicking and marching and increase the number of seconds for each.

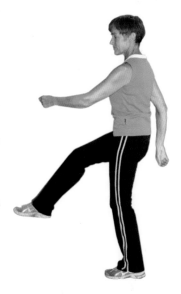

5. TRAVELLING SIDE SQUATS

1. Start with your feet hip-width apart
2. Squat one leg to the side and then travel the other leg in the same direction to stand upright
3. Repeat 4 times moving to the right and 4 times moving back to the left
4. Keep your hips facing forwards
5. Take care not to squat too deeply – maintain a 90-degree angle at the knees
6. Perform for 1–2 minutes

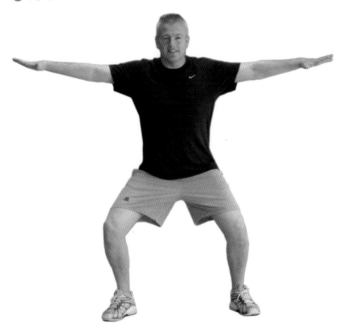

Cardio exercises can help tone the muscles of the lower body, release muscle tension and maintain a healthy body weight.

GET STRONG!

You can perform these exercises after you have finished the cardiovascular exercises if you feel like a longer workout. As usual, it is essential to perform five minutes of the warm-up before trying these exercises. When you have finished, stretch all the muscles while you are nice and warm. Correct breathing is very important: the main thing is not to hold your breath. Ideally, you should breathe out on the effort – the lifting phase of the movement – and breathe in on the lowering phase of the exercise.

1. DEAD-LIFT WITH WEIGHTS

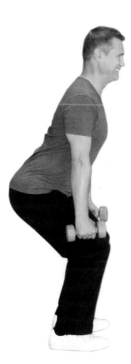

1 Stand upright with your feet hip-width apart

2 Bend at the knees and hips – but don't curve your back – as though you are reaching to lift something from the floor

3 Return to an upright position by straightening your knees and hips and leading with your shoulders

4 Push your buttocks backwards and don't let your knees travel too far forwards

5 Your bottom should be higher than your knees when bending

6 Look forwards and slightly upwards

7 If the exercise feels easy, try lifting a small weight from the floor

8 Start with 8 repetitions and gradually build up to 16–24

Note: You should use this action when lifting any object from the floor.

2. UPRIGHT ROW WITH WEIGHTS

1 Maintain an upright posture with your knees slightly bent, feet hip-width apart

2 Lift up the dumbbells to chest level, keeping them close to your body

3 Lower them down under control

4 Start with 8 repetitions and gradually build up to 16–24

Note: if you don't have dumbbells you can use baked beans or water bottles

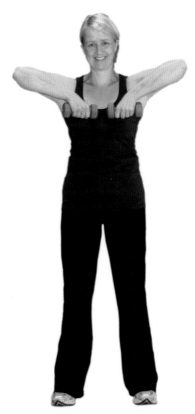

3. SIT-UPS/CURL-UPS

1. Lie on your back with your knees bent and your feet firmly on the floor
2. Place your hands on your thighs
3. Engage your abdominal muscles by pulling in your tummy
4. Use your tummy muscles to curl your shoulders and chest off the floor
5. Lift as far as is comfortable, but without lifting your lower back off the floor
6. Lower yourself down under control
7. Keep your neck relaxed throughout and look forwards
8. Start with 8 repetitions and gradually build up to 16–20

Note: you can make this harder by placing your hands across your chest or at the sides of your head – don't pull at your head as you lift up though.

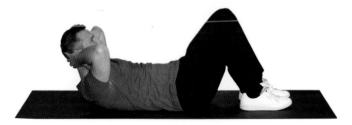

These activities can help tone and shape the muscles. They also provide a release from any tension and improve the posture. Remember not to force the movement and stop if it becomes painful. Don't give up though – after just a few attempts you will find each movement much easier.

4. BACK EXTENSIONS

1. Lie face down on the floor and rest your hands at your side on the floor
2. Engage your abdominals lightly and contract your back muscles
3. Raise your chest away from the floor, keeping your neck in line with the rest of your spine
4. Lower back down to the floor slowly
5. Start with 8 repetitions and gradually build up to 16–20

Note: you can also put your hands on your buttocks or at the sides of your head to make this harder

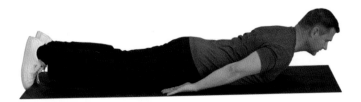

I used to be one of those people who was just 'too busy': too busy to see friends or take a holiday, too busy even to watch my daughter in her school play. I felt stressed all the time and wondered how everyone else managed to cope. Then my wife gave me a gym membership and asked me to try it for a month. Unexpectedly I found that instead of using up my valuable time, it had the opposite effect: it gave me a place to channel my frustration and helped improve my mood. I had better concentration in the office and a better attitude out of it – and what's more, I realised I never wanted to miss another school play ever again.

Paul, aged 36

5. PRESS-UPS

❶ Take up a full plank position with your body straight, supported on your arms and toes

❷ Your hands should be a shoulder width and a half apart

❸ Make sure that your shoulders are further forward than the hands

❹ Engage your abdominals

❺ Bend your elbows to lower your chest towards the wall or floor

❻ Extend your elbows to return to the start position

❼ Keep your elbows unlocked

❽ Start with 8 repetitions and gradually build up to 16–20

Note: you can rest whenever you need to – press-ups are hard! If you prefer, you can do a slightly easier version with your knees bent and resting on the floor, or you can take up a standing position and do press-ups against a wall.

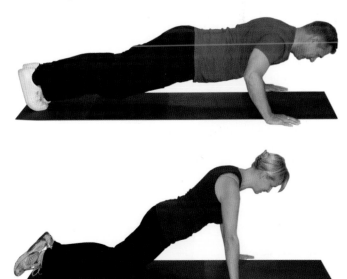

6. CALF RAISE

1 Stand with your feet hip-width apart and engage your abdominals
2 Rest your hands lightly on a chair back if you need support
3 Rise onto the balls of your feet, lifting your heels from the floor
4 Lower your heels under control
5 Keep your knee joints unlocked
6 Start with 8–12 repetitions and gradually build up to 16–24

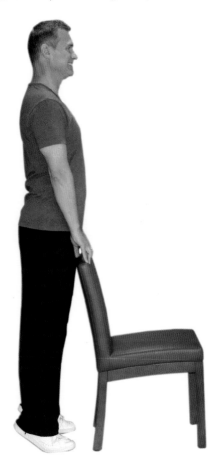

7. BICEPS CURL WITH WEIGHTS

❶ Stand with your feet hip-width apart and engage your abdominals
❷ Fix your elbows in to the sides of your body
❸ Raise the dumbbells in an arc-like motion towards your chest
❹ Lower them under control without locking your elbows
❺ Keep your wrists fixed and straight
❻ Your lower arms should be the only body parts moving
❼ Start with 8–12 repetitions and gradually build up to 16–24

Note: if you do not have dumbbells, use a can of baked beans

OUTER-THIGH RAISES

❶ Lie on one side, engage your abdominals and bend the bottom knee to assist balance
❷ Raise and lower your top leg slowly
❸ Keep your hips facing forwards as you lift your leg up
❹ When the exercise feels easy, you can rest and then perform another set
❺ Start with 8–12 repetitions and gradually build up to 16–24

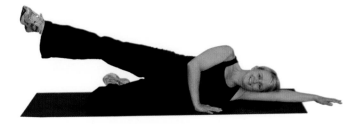

INNER-THIGH RAISES

1. Lie on one side and bend your top knee across your body to rest it on the floor
2. Raise and lower your bottom leg slowly
3. Lift your leg without moving your waist or rolling your hips backwards
4. Start with 8–12 repetitions and gradually build up to 16–24

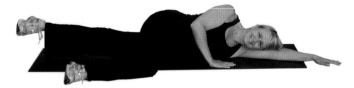

Thank you for reading

We hope you feel inspired by this book to exercise a little more, and have realised how simple it can be. Whether you give yourself ten minutes of desk-relief exercises at work, or plan to put on some music and work your way through a half-hour cardio routine, you will start to feel the benefits almost at once.

But exercise at home isn't for everyone. Some people prefer to get out of the house, into the fresh air or simply want some company. You can do some of these exercises as you walk or jog around the park – just make sure you feel nicely warm beforehand.

Or maybe you prefer a completely different option? Turn over the page for some of our favourite suggestions on pages 96 onwards.

Now go and enjoy yourself!

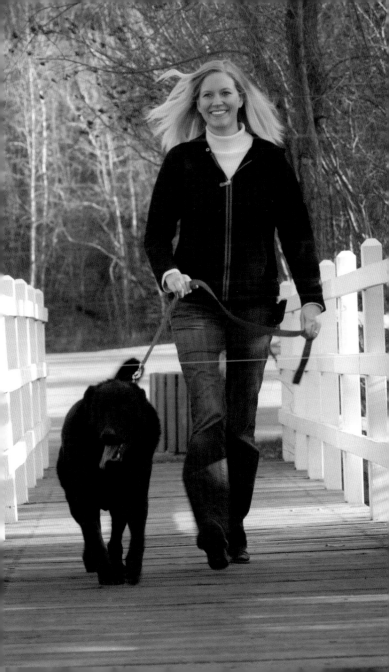

>> Get out and about!

There are lots of forms of exercise that you can do outdoors: walking, climbing, Tai Chi, running, cycling, circuit training, rambling and so on. There's also lots of evidence to suggest that exercising outdoors can have positive results for our mental health.

Getting out into the natural world helps us to recharge and refocus. The natural environment provides an escape for the brain, from some of our dull daily routines, allowing us to relax. There's even some evidence to show that looking at stunning views can actually lower our blood pressure.

While jogging, running and walking are great ways to improve cardiovascular fitness – to keep our hearts and lungs strong – they are also great ways to exercise away stress in the large muscles of the legs, which are activated ready to run during times of stress.

My doctor told me I should start being more active to help lower my blood pressure and manage my weight. He said this would help me to manage my stress levels too, so I joined a local walking group and it has made a big difference. I have met lots of new people and have progressed to a more advanced walking group.

I haven't lost loads of weight, but I feel so much better and so much more in control. The last time I visited my doctor, my blood pressure was lower, so I am chuffed! I am even considering training to become a walk leader now. I would like to help others who are in same boat as I was – up xxxx creek without a paddle! Well, I got my paddle back.

Owen, age 55

>> Walking

> If I could not walk far and fast, I think I
> should just explode and perish.
>
> **Charles Dickens**

Not everyone enjoys going for a jog or a run, but most of us can get
some pleasure out of walking. Aside from the obvious health benefits –
it's good for our heart and lungs and can help ease the build-up of
tension in our muscles – walking is good for us mentally, too. Many
people find that it provides the perfect opportunity to think through
problems and resolve them. The very act of moving, of getting away
from it all, and of breathing deeply because of the physical exertion, can
have a positive effect.

One really good thing about walking is that it's accessible to everyone, at
any level of fitness. And it can also be made to fit any amount of time
you may have: you can walk for fifteen minutes at lunchtime, walk your
kids to school or go for a ten-mile trek in the countryside – it's all good
for you! It can be a solitary pleasure and a time for peaceful
contemplation, or a social activity. Walking with friends is a great
pick-me-up, and can be combined with other pleasures such as visiting
a National Trust property or having a pub lunch.

If you want company on your walk there are plenty of groups you can
join: there are organised sight-seeing walks in most cities; you can
contact a group like the Ramblers; or you can look out for nature walks
in your local area.

Get some fresh air

The easiest way to start is to go for a brisk walk outdoors once a
week for an hour or so. Take time to look at the scenery, watch
birds, feel the fresh air on your face and in your lungs and enjoy
the sense of space.

>> Swimming

Water is a naturally relaxing environment and swimming is a great way to reduce stress. It promotes the circulation of blood and gets rid of any unused energy and mental tension. The pressure of water provides a massaging effect, and its buoyancy automatically reduces some of the physical stress on the body. This makes it a good option if you have joint problems or a low level of fitness, and want to steer clear of high-impact exercises.

There is also some evidence to suggest that immersion in water will calm the part of the nervous system that speeds up during times of stress. This means there are real benefits for your state of mind, even as you tone your body and improve your cardiovascular fitness.

If you aren't a good swimmer then consider taking classes at your local pool – it's never too late to start. Or you could opt for an aqua aerobics class. These are a fun way to exercise, with a trained instructor and a relaxing, non-competitive environment.

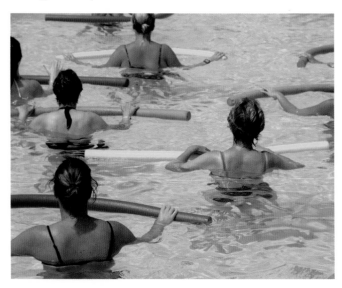

>> Dancing

Dance is a cardiovascular activity with many health benefits. There are so many types of dance that there's really something for everyone: from Ballroom to Tango, Salsa to Jive, a dance class is a great way to get yourself moving and have fun in the process. It's also a very sociable activity and a great way to break down barriers.

If you're not quite ready to dance in public, then all you have to do is clear some space, put on some music and move. There are no rules – anything goes! Whether you've just come home from work, are getting ready to go out or are dancing round the house while doing the dusting, it'll give your mood an instant lift.

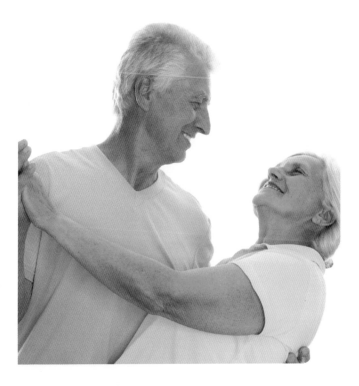

>> Yoga

Yoga is a form of exercise that increases flexibility and promotes strength and balance. Some classes can be quite strenuous while others focus on gentle movements and breathing techniques. If you're interested in taking a class there are usually plenty of options, but try to speak to the instructor and find out if this is the right one for you.

Many people find that yoga not only gives them a greater level of strength and suppleness, but that is also helps them relax and focus. This makes it incredibly beneficial if you have a stressful lifestyle. Another advantage is that yoga can be practised in your own home – all you need is a mat and some loose-fitting clothing. People who start learning yoga as beginners soon feel ready to practise on their own. It is a great tool for taking control and learning to relax.

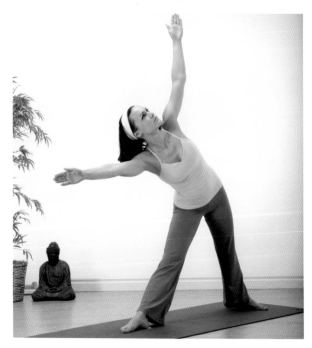

'My mum is 65 years old. She walks her dog every day, shops and cleans for her older brothers and sisters and manages my garden as well as her own. I am always amazed at how this woman climbs ladders, washes windows and chops down trees!

My dad, who is now 78, became very inactive shortly after retiring. He sat watching TV and having tea made for him – he just did not move much. Then, at age of 72, one of life's bombshells hit him: his marriage broke down and he had to move into sheltered housing. He went to the GP because he was feeling depressed and his doctor prescribed some medication. More importantly, though, he advised my father to start exercising.

Dad joined the local gym, which offered a special membership fee for senior members. He now goes to the gym every day and has a circle of friends (all the young mums – they get on like a house on fire!) He tells me, 'I don't push myself. I have 30 minutes on the rower, then 30 minutes on the treadmill, then I do some weights.' I dread to think what he would be doing if he did push himself! Last year he proudly showed me the gym newsletter: he was 'member of the month'.

Dad still gets the blues sometimes – when he thinks that life 'has not turned out the way it should have' – but he knows that going to the gym has made a big difference for him. I've taken a leaf out of his book too.'

Jonathon, aged 55

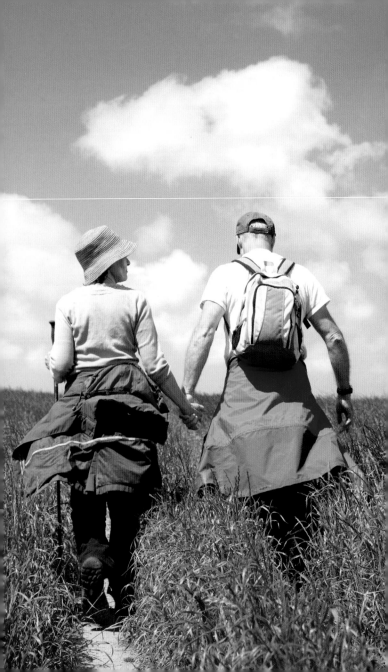

appendices

>> Appendix 1: Resource list

What are the resources in your life, and how are you using them? Are there other resources you can discover that you aren't making the most of?

Resource	How I use it

>> Appendix 2: Activity Log

This can help you to monitor and build your activity levels.

- Start by writing down your current activity levels
- Write down one small change you would like to make to your activity levels on one day
- Make that change and monitor your progress
- When you feel ready, progressively add in more changes on more days

Day / Date	6am–8am	8am–10am	10am–12noon	12noon–2pm	2pm–4pm	4pm–6pm	6pm–8pm	8pm–10pm
Example	Walk to station	Desk exercises		Go for a walk in lunch hour		Walk home from station	Pilates class or swimming	
Monday								
Tuesday								

Day / Date	6am–8am	8am–10am	10am–12noon	12noon–2pm	2pm–4pm	4pm–6pm	6pm–8pm	8pm–10pm
Wednesday								
Thursday								
Friday								
Saturday								
Sunday								

>> Appendix 3: Food and mood diary

You can use a food diary to monitor and make changes to your eating patterns. You can also use the diary to make a note of how your eating affects your mood. This can then help you to look at other strategies you can use to improve your mood and manage your eating.

- Start by writing down everything you eat and drink for one or two days
- Write down one small change you would like to make to your eating habits on one day
- Make that change and monitor your progress
- When you feel ready, progressively build in more changes on more days

Day/Date	Breakfast	Mid-morning snack	Lunch	Mid-afternoon snack	Dinner	Evening snack
Example						
Food	Skipped breakfast Cup of coffee	2 cups of coffee and biscuits	Sardines on toast and coffee	Chocolate bar and 2 cups of coffee	2 glasses of wine Spaghetti Bolognese	

Day/Date	Breakfast	Mid-morning snack	Lunch	Mid-afternoon snack	Dinner	Evening snack
Example						
Mood	Stressed – woke up late	Tired		Angry at boss for giving me another job to finish. Knew I would finish work late again!	Relieved to be home	Tired
Change I would like to make		Take some fruit to eat at break			Drink a glass of water and drink wine after dinner, not before	

>> **Appendix 4: Relaxation script**

- Sit or lie in a comfortable position.
- Allow your body to relax and lengthen.
- Allow the muscles to soften.
- Focus your awareness on your breathing.
- Notice the depth and pace of your breathing.
- Allow your breath to become slower, softer and deeper.
- Take your mind's awareness to your body, starting with the feet.
- Spread and separate your toes, feeling the tension in the feet.
- Flex your toes towards your knees, feeling the tension in the lower leg.
- Stay aware of the tension, breathe steadily in and out.
- Then let the toes and feet relax, let go of any tension in the lower legs.
- Be still and breathe softly and deeply.
- Take your mind's awareness to the thigh muscles.
- Allow the muscles at the front of the thigh to tighten without locking the knee.
- Tighten the muscles at the back of the thigh.
- Squeeze the buttocks tight.
- Stay aware of the tension in the thighs and buttocks, breathe steadily in and out.
- Then let the thigh and buttock muscles relax.
- Feel the hip joint open and soften.
- Feel the whole of the legs relax and soften.
- Be still and breathe softly and deeply.
- Focus your mind's awareness on the abdomen.
- Draw the abdominal muscles in tightly towards your back bone.
- Feel the sides of the abdomen draw in tight.
- Feel the muscles of the lower back tighten.
- Stay aware of the tension, experience the feeling of a corset tightening around the centre of the body, breathe steadily in and out.
- Then release the tension in these muscles and feel the centre of the body relax and let go.
- Be still and breathe softly and deeply.

- Focus your awareness on the shoulders and upper back.
- Squeeze the shoulders towards the ears.
- Feel the tension increase in the muscles of the upper back and the back of the neck, breathe steadily in and out.
- Then allow the muscles to let go and release.
- Lengthen the ears away from the shoulder.
- Feel the chin tucking towards the body.
- Feel the muscles in-between the shoulder blades drawing downwards and tightening.
- Stay aware of the tension, breathe steadily in and out.
- Then release the tension in these muscles, allow the body to let go.
- Be still and breathe softly and deeply.
- Focus your awareness on the muscles of the arms.
- Extend the arms and tense all the muscles in the upper and lower arms, breathe steadily in and out.
- Clench the fist to increase the tension.
- Stay aware of the tension, breathing steadily in and out.
- Then allow the muscles to release and let go.
- Spread the fingers and open up the hands.
- Extend the fingers as far away from the shoulders as you can.
- Stay aware of the tension in the muscles of the hands and arms, breathe steadily in and out.
- Then release and let go and allow the arms to soften and relax.
- Allow the body to be still, breathe slowly and deeply.
- Focus your mind's awareness on the face and head.
- Open your mouth wide and feel the tension around the mouth and jaw.
- Stay aware of the tension, breathe steadily in and out.
- Then release and let go, allow the jaw to relax, wiggle the jaw a little.
- Stick out your tongue, then allow it to relax back into your mouth.
- Feel the tongue soften and the mouth and jaw relax, breathe steadily in and out.
- Wiggle your nose and then release.
- Feel the eye sockets opening and then release.

Move the muscles in the forehead, then allow them to soften and relax.

- Let the body sink deeper and relax further.
- Any tension just easing away.
- Tighten the whole body one last time, extending your head and toes and fingers as far away from each other as you can.
- Release and let go, allow yourself to sigh.
- Take your mind's awareness back to your breathing.
- Focus on slower, deeper breathing.
- Allow your body to be still and silent.
- With every breath allow the body to relax further.
- Allow a feeling of relaxation and calm to spread through your whole body.

bibliography

ACSM (2005) 7th edition. *ACSM's Guidelines for Exercise Testing and Prescription*. USA. Lippincott, Williams & Wilkins.

Benson, H, MD (1975). *The Relaxation Response*. New York. Avon books.

Biddle, S, Fox, K & Boutcher, S (2000) Eds. *Physical Activity and Psychological Well-Being*. London and New York. Routledge.

Bird, W (2007). 'Natural Thinking: A Report for the Royal Society for the Protection of Birds Investigating the Links Between the Natural Environment, Biodiversity and Mental Health'. Available from www.rspb.org.uk.

Borg G (1998). *Perceived Exertion and Pain Scales*. USA. Human Kinetics.

British National Formulary (2005). 'Joint National Formulary Committee. British National Formulary. (50 ed)'. London. British Medical Association and Royal Pharmaceutical Society of Great Britain. Available from: www.bnf.org.uk

British Nutrition Foundation (2005). 'Balance of Good Health'. Available from: www.nutrition.org.uk.

Davison, G & Neale, J (2001) 8th edition. *Abnormal Psychology*. USA. John Wiley & Sons.

Department of Health (2004). 'At Least Five a Week: Evidence on the Impact of Physical Activity and Its Relationship to Health. A report from the Chief Medical Officer'. London. Department of Health.

Department of Health (2004). 'Choosing Health: Making Healthier Choices Easier'. London. Department of Health.

Durstine, L J & Moore, G (2003) 2nd edition. *ACSM's Exercise Management for Persons with Chronic Diseases and Disabilities*. USA. Human Kinetics.

Feltham, C & Horton, I (2000) Eds. *Handbook of Counselling and Psychotherapy*. UK. Sage publications.

Fernando, S (1988). *Race and Culture in Psychiatry*. London. Croom Helm.

Gross, R & McIlveen, R (1998). *Psychology: A New Introduction*. London. Hodder & Stoughton.

Halliwell, E (2005). 'UP and Running? Exercise Therapy and the Treatment of Mild or Moderate Depression in Primary Care'. UK. Available from: www.mentalhealth.org.uk.

Health and Safety Executive (2005). 'Stress Related and Psychological Disorders'. UK. Available from: www.hse.gov.uk.

Hendrix, M (1994). 'Anxiety Disorders'. USA. Available from: www.nimh.nih.gov.

Lago, C & Thompson, J (2003). *Race, Culture and Counselling*. Berkshire. Open University Press.

Lawrence, D (2004) 2nd edition. *The Complete Guide to Exercise in Water*. London. A&C Black.

Lawrence, D (2004) 2nd edition. *The Complete Guide to Exercise to Music*. London. A&C Black.

Lawrence, D (2005). *The Complete Guide to Exercising Away Stress*. London. A&C Black.

Lawrence, D & Barnett, L (2006). *GP referral Schemes*. London. A&C Black.

Mindell, A (1995). *Sitting in the Fire: Large Group Transformation Using Conflict and Diversity*. USA. Lao Tse Press.

Raistrick, D, Hodgson, R & Ritson, B (1999). *Tackling Alcohol Together*. Free Association Books.

Rogers, C & Stevens, B (1967). *Person To Person: The Problem of Being Human*. USA. Real People Press.

Spada, M (2006). *Overcoming Problem Drinking*. London. Robinson Publishing.

find out more

Al-Anon Family Groups UK and Eire
www.al-anonuk.org.uk

Alcoholics Anonymous
www.alcoholics-anonymous.org.uk
Tel: 0845 769 7555

Alcohol Concern
www.alcoholconcern.org.uk

Alcohol – know your units
www.rcpsych.ac.uk/www.units.nhs.uk

BACP (British Association of Counselling and Psychotherapy)
www.bacp.co.uk

Change4life
www.change4life.com

Cruse Bereavement Care
www.crusebereavementcare.org.uk/AboutGrief.html